Trauma- and Stressor-Related Disorders

A HANDBOOK FOR CLINICIANS

Trauma- and Stressor-Related Disorders

A HANDBOOK FOR CLINICIANS

Edited by

Patricia R. Casey, M.D., F.R.C.Psych.

James J. Strain, M.D.

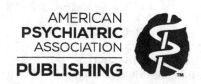

AMERICAN
PSYCHIATRIC
ASSOCIATION
PUBLISHING

If you wish to buy 50 or more copies of the same title, please go to www.appi.org/special-discounts for more information.

Copyright © 2016 American Psychiatric Association Publishing

Manufactured in the United States of America on acid-free paper

19 18 17 16 15   5 4 3 2 1
First Edition

Typeset in Minion Pro and Trade Gothic LT Std.

American Psychiatric Association Publishing
1000 Wilson Boulevard
Arlington, VA 22209-3901
www.appi.org

Library of Congress Cataloging-in-Publication Data
Trauma- and stressor-related disorders: a handbook for clinicians / edited by Patricia R. Casey, James J. Strain.
    p. ; cm.
Includes bibliographical references and index.
ISBN 978-1-58562-505-5 (pb : alk. paper)
I. Casey, Patricia R., editor. II. Strain, James J., 1933–, editor.
  [DNLM: 1. Stress Disorders, Traumatic—diagnosis. 2. Stress Disorders, Traumatic—therapy. 3. Adjustment Disorders—diagnosis. 4. Adjustment Disorders—therapy. WM 172.5]
RC552.T7
616.85'21—dc23
                                  2015031473

British Library Cataloguing in Publication Data
A CIP record is available from the British Library.

Contents

Contributors

Richard A. Bryant, Ph.D.
Scientia Professor and NHMRC Senior Principal Research Fellow, School of Psychology, University of New South Wales, Sydney, New South Wales, Australia

Patricia R. Casey, M.D., F.R.C.Psych.
Professor of Psychiatry, University College Dublin, and Consultant Psychiatrist, Misericordiae University Hospital, Dublin, Ireland

Dennis S. Charney, M.D.
Dean, Icahn School of Medicine at Mount Sinai, and Professor, Departments of Psychiatry, Neuroscience, and Pharmacology and Systems Therapeutics, Icahn School of Medicine at Mount Sinai, New York, New York

Colleen E. Gribbin, M.A.
Program Manager, Center for Complicated Grief, and Project Coordinator, Kenworthy Projects, Columbia University School of Social Work, New York, New York

Brian M. Iacoviello, Ph.D.
Assistant Professor, Department of Psychiatry, Icahn School of Medicine at Mount Sinai, New York, New York

Amy Lehrner, Ph.D.
Clinical Psychologist, James J. Peters Veterans Affairs Medical Center, Bronx, New York, and Assistant Professor, Department of Psychiatry, Icahn School of Medicine at Mount Sinai, New York, New York

Andreas Maercker, M.D., Ph.D.
Professor of Psychology, Department of Psychology, University of Zurich, Zurich, Switzerland

Axel Perkonigg, Ph.D.
Scientific Assistant, Department of Psychology, University of Zurich, Zurich, Switzerland

Laura C. Pratchett, Psy.D.
Clinical Psychologist, James J. Peters Veterans Affairs Medical Center, Bronx, New York, and Assistant Clinical Professor, Department of Psychiatry, Icahn School of Medicine at Mount Sinai, New York, New York

Phillip J. Resnick, M.D.
Professor of Psychiatry, Case Western Reserve University School of Medicine, Cleveland, Ohio

M. Katherine Shear, M.D.
Marion E. Kenworthy Professor of Psychiatry in Social Work, Columbia University School of Social Work and Columbia University College of Physicians and Surgeons, New York, New York

David Spiegel, M.D.
Jack, Lulu & Sam Willson Professor and Associate Chair, Department of Psychiatry and Behavioral Sciences, Stanford University School of Medicine, Stanford, California

James J. Strain, M.D.
Professor of Psychiatry and Professor of Medical Education and Master Teacher, Icahn School of Medicine at Mount Sinai, New York, New York

Peter Tyrer, M.D.
Professor of Community Psychiatry, Centre for Mental Health, Imperial College, London, UK

Henry C. Weinstein, M.D.
Clinical Professor of Psychiatry, Department of Psychiatry, New York University School of Medicine, New York, New York

Rachel Yehuda, Ph.D.
Mental Health Patient Care Center Director, James J. Peters Veterans Affairs Medical Center, Bronx, New York, and Professor, Department of Psychiatry, Icahn School of Medicine at Mount Sinai, New York, New York

DISCLOSURE OF INTERESTS

The following contributor to this book has indicated a financial interest in or other affiliation with a commercial supporter, a manufacturer of a commercial product, a provider of a commercial service, a nongovernmental organization, and/or a government agency, as listed below:

M. Katherine Shear, M.D.   *Royalties:* Guilford Press

The following contributors have indicated that they have no financial interests or other affiliations that represent or could appear to represent a competing interest with their contributions to this book:

Patricia R. Casey, M.D., F.R.C.Psych., Brian M. Iacoviello, Ph.D., Amy Lehrner, Ph.D., Andreas Maercker, M.D., Ph.D., Laura C. Pratchett, Psy.D., David Spiegel, M.D., James J. Strain, M.D., Peter Tyrer, M.D., Rachel Yehuda, Ph.D.

Foreword

THIS MARVELOUS, comprehensive book that Drs. Patricia Casey and James Strain and have put together helps clinicians deal with issues that focus on trauma- and stressor-related disorders. Distinguishing between normal and pathological responses has long been a challenge for people in the field of psychiatric medicine. When is grief, a pervasive phenomenon, so severe so as to be considered pathological? When is therapeutic intervention indicated? Is there a neurobiological similarity between minor disorders and major disability? Could this facilitate identification of a biological marker for dysfunction in an early state? Generating guidelines for diagnosis to promote a conceptual framework to approaching these challenges is important.

There are no tests to demonstrate psychiatric or adjustment disorders. As clinicians, we use the best tools and techniques we have in terms of observation of phenomenology; diagnostic categories, which the field updates regularly; and clinical judgment. DSM-5 and ICD-11 have produced organizing frameworks for these disorders, and the chapter authors have carefully elaborated the differences to help guide readers. They recognize the value from ongoing research that will foster greater classification. Simultaneously, these issues have enormous relevance for medical-legal aspects.

Enduring the loss of important individuals, such as family and friends, has a major impact on individuals. The clinician struggles to decide when to intervene. Sometimes it is wiser to leave the individual alone and let time heal. Sometimes, despite the fact that grief in itself is not pathological, outside assistance is warranted. Often, the impact on the grieving family or friends does not immediately manifest because people have a tendency to conceal hurt.

The tremendous impact of posttraumatic stress disorders on veterans is obvious. Working to find optimal treatments of these disorders and recognizing their complexity and seriousness is critical for clinicians.

Drs. Casey and Strain are long-standing, highly knowledgeable clinical academics in the arena of trauma- and stressor-related disorders, and this book provides informed advice for clinicians dealing with this set of issues. Readers will be well served and will enjoy this book, getting the benefit of authoritative advice and, as a result, improving their efforts in dealing with patients, families, and professionals who are challenged by these disorders. This volume provides an enriching and rewarding adventure into the understanding of these most interesting psychological states.

Herbert Pardes, M.D.
Executive Vice Chairman of the Board of Trustees of
New York-Presbyterian University Hospital of Columbia and Cornell
Former Director of the National Institutes of Mental Health
Former President of the American Psychiatric Association
Former Dean and Chair of Psychiatry, Columbia-Presbyterian School of Medicine

Preface

THE CAUSAL role of stress and trauma in the etiology of some psychiatric disorders has long been recognized. In DSM-5 (American Psychiatric Association 2013), a new diagnostic class termed *trauma- and stressor-related disorders* has been added to include, among other disorders, adjustment disorders (ADs), acute stress disorder (ASD), and posttraumatic stress disorder (PTSD). The trauma- and stressor-related disorders are grouped together because each of them requires a stressor or traumatic stressor for diagnosis. In no other set of DSM-5 diagnoses is a stressor required as an etiological agent, although stress may be involved with the precipitation or occurrence of some disorders (e.g., major depressive disorder). This dimension of the diagnosis—a stressor as an etiological agent—also adds considerable controversy to these diagnoses: First, when is an event a stressor to an individual, and furthermore, when is the stressor considered traumatic? Second, what influence does the culture of the patient exact on the experience of an event as a stressor? The DSM-5 work group considering these disorders worked long and hard to define when a stressor is indeed a stressor. However, deciding when an event is a stressor and, in some cases, when a stressor is indeed traumatic remains quite subjective.

The inclusion of ADs in the trauma- and stressor-related grouping is a landmark change. Underresearched and arguably underdiagnosed, AD was previously orphaned in its own category. In DSM-IV (American Psychiatric Association 1994), it had its own placement and was not included in the anxiety disorder category. The move into a grouping that is well researched and has high relevance may have the domino effect of stimulating interest in ADs.

A work that deals with trauma- and stressor-related disorders is especially challenging because it poses many questions, some of a philosophical nature: How can abnormal reactions to events be distinguished from those that are appropriate? What would constitute a normal reaction to witnessing a massacre or to losing a loved one to murder? How can some of these disorders be distinguished from each other and from normal reactions? For example, is a person

with terminal cancer who is constantly distressed reacting normally or abnormally, and if the latter, does he or she have major depressive disorder or AD?
How do therapists deal with the limitations of the diagnostic process in psychiatry that is based exclusively on descriptive psychopathology? Many of the
symptoms are heterogeneous, and the same diagnosis can be made in people
with markedly differing symptom patterns. What are the clinical implications of
these differences in symptoms that are associated with the same diagnosis, and
can or should they be resolved?

The continuing and recent developments regarding the neurobiology of
stress provided further impetus for the writing of this volume. Although most
highly developed for the PTSD diagnosis, neurobiology research has long been a
focus for stress researchers. As neurobiological understanding and underpinnings of psychiatric disorders are unfolding, we hope that such research will elu-
cidate biological mechanisms for other stress disorders as well. Considerations
include, for example, whether AD with depressed mood has any correlation with
the neurobiological characteristics observed with major depressive disorder,
whether AD with anxiety correlates with those findings in generalized anxiety
disorder, and so on. It is an exciting era in psychiatry as we strive to understand
the neurobiological mechanisms underlying mental disorders.

In DSM-5, PTSD has been refined and the definition of what constitutes a
traumatic event clarified. Other features that were part of the DSM-IV diagnosis,
such as helplessness, intense fear, and horror, have been removed from Criterion
A because they had low predictive validity in determining who later develops
PTSD in response to a trauma. The core features have now been extended to include a cluster with negative alterations in cognitions and mood, in addition to
the previously included heightened arousal, reexperiencing of the event, and
avoidance. Two subtypes—preschool subtype (for ages 6 years and younger)
and PTSD with dissociative symptoms—are additions. ASD has also been
changed in DSM-5, with removal of the person's subjective response to the
trauma from the criteria. Reactive attachment disorder has been relocated from
other disorders of infancy, childhood, or adolescence in DSM-IV to the trauma-
and stressor-related disorders in DSM-5 because this disorder is the result of
social neglect or other situations that limit a young child's opportunity to form
selective attachments, causing withdrawal, fear, sadness, and failure to seek
comfort or to respond when it is offered. This disorder is not discussed in this
book, which deals only with adult disorders. Disinhibited social engagement
disorder is also not discussed in this book because the disorder is nearly always
associated with children and youth.

The position of abnormal grief (persistent complex bereavement disorder)
in DSM-5 has been a source of controversy. In DSM-IV, bereavement was not
regarded as a specific disorder but instead was assigned a V code (i.e., it was
listed as a condition that may be a focus of clinical attention). In DSM-IV, it was

recognized that at times bereavement presents with symptoms of major depression, and therefore features that distinguish one from the other were provided. It was anticipated by the DSM-5 work group that prolonged grief disorder would be a fully recognized syndrome in DSM-5. This did not happen, however, and instead persistent complex bereavement disorder was included in the category with other specified trauma- and stressor-related disorders, which also includes 1) adjustment-like disorders with delayed onset of symptoms that occur more than 3 months after the stressor, 2) adjustment-like disorders with prolonged duration of more than 6 months without prolonged duration of stressor, 3) *ataque de nervios,* and 4) other cultural syndromes. Unfortunately, these four entities and persistent complex bereavement disorder all employ the same code—309.89 (F43.8)—and therefore cannot be differentiated for clinical or research purposes.

Our own particular interest in ADs, coupled with the major revisions to the DSM trauma- and stressor-related disorder categories summarized above, prompted us to develop this book, which for the first time has brought together all the conditions now classified in this DSM-5 group. To assist us in our task, we approached international experts in these topics. The reaction to our proposal was most heartening, and we present the fruits of the labors of all our contributors.

As practicing clinicians, albeit with a strong research background, our starting point was that the work should first and foremost be clinically relevant. For this reason we have included case vignettes, useful Web sites, and a limited number of references. However, we believe that the controversies posed with particular prominence in this group of disorders could not be ignored and that discussion of them will enrich clinical practice as well as academic acumen. Accordingly, we have attempted to address these controversies in some of the earlier chapters and within other chapters where appropriate.

We hope that these aspirations have been achieved and that *Trauma- and Stressor-Related Disorders: A Handbook for Clinicians* will assist, support, and stimulate clinicians in their day-to-day work. Our patients deserve no less.

James J. Strain, M.D.
Patricia R. Casey, M.D., F.R.C.Psych.

REFERENCES

American Psychiatric Association: Diagnostic and Statistical Manual of Mental Disorders, 4th Edition. Washington, DC, American Psychiatric Association, 1994

American Psychiatric Association: Diagnostic and Statistical Manual of Mental Disorders, 5th Edition, Arlington, VA, American Psychiatric Association 2013

Acknowledgments

I WANT to say a special word of thanks to my coeditor and coauthor, Dr. Jim Strain, for his unstinting commitment to our work and for his generous and gentlemanly approach to resolving the hurdles that we faced from time to time.

I want to thank all the contributors, who rose to the challenge of producing a book that combines academic and clinical perspectives on the trauma- and stressor-related disorders. The remarkable interest and commitment shown by Dr. Robert Hales, Mr. John McDuffie, and Ms. Bessie Jones since our first approaching American Psychiatric Association Publishing has been a huge encouragement to us, and we are deeply grateful. It has been a pleasure working with them and their accomplished and professional support team.

Patricia R. Casey, M.D., F.R.C.Psych.

I wish to acknowledge the many colleagues who have contributed to this volume and made it a reality. The depth of their knowledge and dedication to their special areas of interest are why we are so proud to have them as colleagues. I would especially like to acknowledge Dr. Patricia Casey as coeditor and coauthor for constantly making positive and helpful contributions to the production of this volume, which she suggested we write. There are many persons at American Psychiatric Association Publishing who have supported us and done their jobs skillfully, including Dr. Robert Hales, Mr. John McDuffie, Ms. Carrie Farnham, and Ms. Bessie Jones.

I would like to acknowledge the constant support of my wife, Dr. Gladys Witt Strain, who has enthusiastically endorsed my many projects. I would like to acknowledge my three sons, Drs. Jay, Jeffrey, and Jamie Strain, who have assisted me over the years in a variety of ways—especially Jay, who has been a working collaborator since he was 14 years old. I would like to highlight the important contribution to my work over the years by Mrs. Cynthia Green Colin, Trustee Emeritus of the Mount Sinai Hospital and School of Medicine. She has generously supported my work with first the Green Fund and now the Malcom Gibbs Fund for more than 35 years, truly allowing many academic efforts to go forward. I would like to acknowledge the many psychosomatic fellows whom I have trained and who have taught me; my mentors, Charles Brenner, T. George Bidder, and Marvin Stein (who provided me a clinical laboratory at the Mount Sinai Hospital and School of Medicine); Thomas Dell, who encouraged me to go into medicine; and Ronald G. Witt, who emphasized the need to be academically disciplined and strive for excellence.

James J. Strain, M.D.

CHAPTER 1

Borderline Between Normal and Pathological Responses

PATRICIA R. CASEY, M.D., F.R.C.PSYCH.

UNTIL THE twentieth century the focus of psychiatry/medicine was on what have broadly been described as the endogenous mental disorders such as schizophrenia, melancholia, mania, and dementia. Emil Kraepelin (1856–1926), Eugen Bleuler (1857–1939), and Kurt Schneider (1887–1967) were the key influences in these early days of psychiatry. The conditions they researched occurred not in response to any external triggers but rather within the individual. This limited emphasis began to change under the influence of Sigmund Freud (1856–1939), who initially (although he later changed his position) identified an exogenous factor, sexual trauma in childhood, as a trigger to neurotic phenomena. Karl Jaspers (1883–1969), a philosopher and psychiatrist and the founder of phenomenology, was the first to recognize that psychological reactions to stressful events could constitute mental disorders (Jaspers 1913/1997). He called them "psychogenic" reactions and identified a clear causal connection with respect to the onset, content, and course of the symptoms.

A further development was the recognition that life stressors could also play a role in triggering the onset of conditions formerly thought to be endogenous, especially depression. This realization culminated in the abandonment in DSM-III (American Psychiatric Association 1980) of concepts such as *reactive* and *endogenous* depression and their replacement by *major depression* as a unitary disorder, with differences based on severity only. DSM-III (pp. 6–7) declared itself to be agnostic about etiology. One of the planks of this perspective was the acceptance that episodes of major depression may be triggered by life events and that they can also occur without any such antecedent. This had begun with the work of Mapother (1926) in Britain and others after him who failed to confirm a binary model of depression (endogenous versus reactive). By the time the revisionists came to work on DSM-III, the absence of empirical support for two types of depression led them to abandon these terms and replace them with a unitary model that they called *major depression*. Hence, major depression is not classified as a stress-induced disorder even though studies suggest that major life events precede the onset in many cases.

ZONES OF RARITY

The distinction between psychiatric disorders distinct from each other and from normality has exercised the most important philosophical and psychiatric minds for decades (Cooper 2013; Kendell and Jablensky 2003; Wakefield 1997). The thinking is that discrete categorical disorders should possess natural boundaries from each other and from normal distress, a perspective that is rooted in the assumption of disease entity. For example, posttraumatic stress disorder (PTSD) should differ from major depression and from generalized anxiety disorder, and each in turn should be distinct from normal distress. The cleavage that separates various diagnostic categories from each other and from normality is called a *zone of rarity*. According to this concept, a clear demarcation should exist between those individuals who are ill and those who are not, with few, if any, in the intermediate zone. This is the approach used in general medicine, where various diseases are recognized and distinguished from others by their symptoms, etiology, pathophysiology, course, and prognosis, and the process involved in each of these domains is termed *validation*. However, although, for example, sickle cell anemia is either present or absent, this binary model does not apply to all medical conditions. For instance, like most common mental illnesses, obesity and hypertension are conditions that exist on a continuum, with cutoffs determining what constitutes illness.

The architects of DSM-III envisaged that over time, the descriptive approach to classification would allow for the validation of the various diagnoses. These would be the foundation for research, mapping onto genetic and psychobiological parameters that would ultimately determine individualized treatments. This vision has not been realized. DSM-5 (American Psychiatric Association 2013) continues to be based largely on descriptive psychopathology, and few of the conditions have been validated. Some researchers and clinicians working in this area have suggested that DSM-5 should include as mental disorders those syndromal categories that have been validated (Stein et al. 2010) on the basis of key measures such as prognostic significance, evidence of psychobiological disruption, or prediction of response to treatment but include the weakly validated conditions in Chapter 11, "ICD-10, ICD-11, and DSM-5," as conditions requiring further research. This arrangement would allow the validated syndromes to be mined for further information on etiology, treatment, and prognosis, while the validity of the others could be further tested.

One of the problems with this conceptualization is that in psychopathology clear demarcations do not exist between various psychiatric conditions, especially the common mental disorders such as major depression, adjustment disorder, and generalized anxiety disorder (Maj 2011). They have "fuzzy boundaries" with multiple interacting causes acting on multiple brain mechanisms (Stein et al. 2013). Some researchers further suggest that conditions such as major depression are not single entities, as is commonly believed, but instead comprise "multiple different constituent conditions with each subset likely to have differing biological, psychological and social causal weightings, varying intrinsic illness trajectories and differential responses to contrasting treatment modalities" (Parker 2014, pp. 458–459). This symptom overlap calls into question the validity of many of the syndromes conventionally regarded as discrete psychiatric disorders (Kendell and Jablensky 2003). The impacts of the failure to identify clear demarcations between different disorders are that definitive diagnosis is difficult and concordance over time is poor. Symptoms of abnormal grief overlap with those of major depression, adjustment disorder overlaps with major depression (Casey et al. 2006), and PTSD symptoms such as intrusive memories may be found in major depression (Reynolds and Brewin 1999).

Equally problematic are attempts to distinguish normality from pathology. It has been assumed that there are qualitative differences between normal sadness and pathological sadness and that their gestalt differs above and beyond the sum total of the depressive symptoms (Helmchen and Linden 2000). These differences have been explored, and the most common description was the experience of lethargy and inability to do things, whether because of tiredness or an inability to summon up effort. Also identified in those with pathological reactions were a feeling of being inhibited and an inability to envisage the future, a sense of detachment from the environment, and physical changes similar to a viral illness (Healy 1993). Additionally, according to Clarke and Kissane (2002), individuals who are sad are able to experience pleasure when distracted from demoralizing thoughts, and they feel inhibited in action by not knowing what to do and by feeling helpless and incompetent, whereas individuals with depression have lost motivation and drive and are unable to act even when an appropriate direction of action is known. Nevertheless, attempts to apply these differentiating features in studies using complex statistical methods to classification have been unsuccessful (Maj 2011).

In DSM, an attempt was made to deal with the absence of clear lines of demarcation by requiring that certain criteria are met before a diagnosis is made. In theory this is appealing, but in reality the distinction between what is normal and what is pathological remains problematic. This has resulted in a tendency to falsely diagnose psychiatric disorder when there is none, which is referred to as the false-positive dilemma (as discussed in the next section, "The False-Positive Dilemma and the DSM Approach").

The consequences of false diagnoses for individuals who do not have mental illness are well recognized. These include the medicalization of ordinary suffering, the use of interventions (pharmacological or psychological) for emotional responses where none are needed because these reactions are self-limiting, the possible stigmatization from being diagnosed with a mental illness, the implications for individuals newly seeking health insurance coverage (because many insurers exclude persons with prior illness), and the change in self-perspective that a person experiences when diagnosed with a psychiatric disorder. Finally, false diagnoses of an illness may inflate prevalence data in epidemiological studies and may increase beliefs about chronicity in individuals experiencing continuing sadness.

THE FALSE-POSITIVE DILEMMA AND THE DSM APPROACH

Historically, the growth of the antipsychiatry movement in the 1950s was a reaction to pathologizing the day-to-day tribulations of life, partly influenced by the psychodynamic school of psychiatry. This concern with overdiagnosis led the architects of DSM-III to address the issue. At that time the debate centered on whether homosexuality was a psychiatric disorder. In response Robert Spitzer (1981) developed an approach to diagnosis that is still used today—the clinically significant distress-impairment criterion, which is discussed in the next section ("The Distress-Impairment Criterion"). Because homosexuality per se was not associated with distress or impairment in functioning, it could not be classified as a disorder (Spitzer 1981).

The issue of false positives is particularly relevant with respect to trauma- and stressor-induced disorders because stressful events in life are part of the human condition and they generate a concomitant emotional reaction. They are ordinarily self-limiting, although some people are afflicted by long-standing or repeated stressors and accompanying demoralization. DSM-IV (American Psychiatric Association 1994) approached the clinical problem of distinguishing normal stress responses from those that are adaptive, stating that the response "must not merely be an expectable and culturally sanctioned response to a particular event, for example, the death of a loved one" (p. xxi). However, "expectable" is vague, and although many individuals experiencing "expectable distress"—for example, after financial ruin—are able to cope, albeit with a sense of disappointment, demoralization, and distress, others become overwrought, develop significant mood disturbance, and try to take their lives. Judging what constitutes a normal or expectable response, in contrast to a pathological one in a particular context, requires wisdom in the absence of any assistance from science. The cudgel has been taken up by Maj (2012), who has called for a refinement of the diagnostic systems (ICD and DSM), arguing that "we may also need a description of ordinary responses to major stressors (such as bereavement, economic ruin, exposure to disaster or war, disruption of family by divorce or separation) as well as to life-cycle transitions (e.g., adolescent emotional turmoil)" (p. 138) so as to end the confusion and uncertainty that exists in this regard.

Symptoms alone are not sufficient to identify a particular disorder in response to a stressful event because distress, anxiety, low mood, and so on are universal features of the human condition in certain circumstances. If symptoms in themselves were indicative of psychiatric illness, then 100% of the population would meet the criteria for some mental disorder. When biomarkers are not present, it is difficult to make sense of these features when people describe them.

The possibility of false positives is not simply theoretical, arising from the inadequacy of the current method of classifying psychiatric diagnoses. It was demonstrated empirically when data from the National Institute of Mental Health's Epidemiologic Catchment Area (ECA) study and the National Comorbidity Survey (NCS) were reanalyzed. The addition of the clinical significance criterion resulted in a reduction in the 1-year prevalence estimates for "any disorder" by 17% in the ECA study and by 32% in the NCS (Narrow et al. 2002). Clearly, the incorporation of clinical significance is helpful in reducing the false-positive rate (as discussed in the next section, "The Distress-Impairment Criterion").

The distinction between pathology and normality is most obviously, but not exclusively, important in relation to adjustment disorders (ADs). These disorders are broadly defined in DSM-5 as stress-related disturbances beginning within 3 months of the onset of a stressor and lasting no longer than 6 months after the stressor or its consequences have ceased. They are characterized by marked distress or significant impairment and must not meet the criteria for another mental disorder. Thus, they are a subthreshold disorder. There are no specific symptom criteria, but there are subtypes marked by depressed mood, anxious symptoms, or disturbance of conduct. In this they are different from the other DSM-5 trauma- and stressor-related disorders, all of which have detailed diagnostic criteria that enable diagnosis, however imperfect these criteria may be.

The problem of distinguishing normal reactions from pathological responses is illustrated in the following case vignette and exemplifies the issue raised by Maj (2012) concerning the need for descriptions of normal responses to major stressors.

Case Vignette

Mr. C was referred to an outpatient clinic because his house had been very badly damaged after a fire due to an electrical problem. The house was vacant at the time, and nobody was injured. Mr. C returned to find the fire department at work putting out the fire. He had another house (ordinarily rented to tenants but vacant at the time) into which he moved while the damaged one was being renovated. When first seen 6 weeks after the event, he was distressed about what had happened. He had required 4 days off from his job as a company manager but was back at work. His work was somewhat affected in that he was at times distracted when thinking about the event, but nobody at work noticed or commented on his distraction except a close friend. Mr. C had no nightmares or flashbacks, and he generally slept well except about 1 night each week when he would recapitulate what happened. His appetite was good, but he often thought about what might have happened if he had been in the house at the time, and he worried about another fire happening in the future. Mr. C's general practitioner wondered if he had PTSD.

The clinician considered several questions: What is a normal reaction to such an event? Was Mr. C's reaction excessive or proportionate to the event? Did he have any symptoms that would clearly distinguish his response from one of the recognized psychiatric disorders that such an event might give rise to— PTSD, ADs, or generalized anxiety disorder? Was he impaired functionally for any period in the aftermath, and if so, was the duration excessive? Could he be regarded as having a subthreshold disorder? The clinician decided that Mr. C did not have any psychiatric disorder and recommended that a hypnotic be taken as needed. When the patient was seen again 3 months later, all his symptoms had resolved apart from continuing general concerns about another fire happening in the future.

The DSM-5 approach to grief and distinguishing it from major depression is a good example of the positive manner in which attempts to distinguish normal reactions from pathological reactions are dealt with in DSM-5, as suggested by Maj (2012). In response to the removal of the bereavement exclusion for major depression, DSM-5 provides a detailed description of the differences between normal grief and severe grief response that is best classified as major depression. This is discussed in greater detail later in this chapter (see "Clinical Judgment").

THE DISTRESS-IMPAIRMENT CRITERION

In attempting to define what psychiatric disorder is, stimulated by a discussion regarding homosexuality, Spitzer (1981) proposed that psychiatric illness, in its manifestation, should be associated with clinically significant distress or impairment in social, occupational, or other important areas of functioning. The centrality of clinically significant distress or impairment in defining psychiatric disorders has been restated in subsequent editions of DSM, although DSM-IV recognized the limitations:

> [I]t must be admitted that no definition adequately specifies precise boundaries for the concept of "mental disorder."… Mental disorders have…been defined by a variety of concepts (e.g., distress, dyscontrol, disadvantage, disability, inflexibility, irrationality, syndromal pattern, etiology, and statistical deviation). Each is a useful indicator for a mental disorder, but none is equivalent to the concept, and different situations call for different definitions. (American Psychiatric Association 1994, p. xxi)

Some authors (e.g., Cooper 2013) argue that DSM-5 has weakened the distress-impairment criterion by altering the wording such that it need not be present in all conditions. In the section "Use of the Manual," DSM-5 now reads, "Mental disorders are *usually* [emphasis added] associated with significant distress or disability in social, occupational, or other important activities" (American Psychiatric Press 2013, p. 20). It remains to be seen in which conditions and in what circumstances this less definitive approach will emerge.

Critics of the DSM system point out that the clinical significance criterion is tautological (Frances 1998) because it is merely saying that symptoms are clinically significant if they are judged to be clinically significant by doctors treating them. No further operationalization of this clinical significance is provided. The decision to consult with a mental health professional might indicate clinical significance. If the fact of seeking help per se were the determining factor, then individuals who are visiting their doctors at the behest of others might not be viewed as having clinically significant symptoms. However, what if frequent consultation is part of a pattern of behavior in which minor symptoms are magnified because of excessive health preoccupations on the part of patients? Alternatively, does the absence of consultation point to the absence of clinical significance such as is often present in those individuals with masked illnesses or those lacking insight? Perhaps an individual is stoic or may believe that his or her doctor is not sufficiently empathic to consider a consultation. Basing this criterion simply on consultation habits would have significant implications for population-based epidemiological studies using lay interviewers who would inevitably have to regard every face-to-face contact with a doctor as clinically significant, thereby potentially inflating the number of false positives.

If, however, both distress due to symptoms and functional impairment were required, this might further strengthen the boundary between normal responses to problems of living and recognized mental disorders. The superior power of functional impairment over symptom severity as a predictor of outcome has been demonstrated (Casey et al. 2004), suggesting that functional impairment warrants serious attention in the assessment of symptoms. Indeed, ICD-10 (World Health Organization 1992) specifies that both symptoms and impairment should be present for a diagnosis of ADs (see Chapter 11). The possible benefits of requiring both social dysfunction and symptoms in separating disorder from normality need further study. Although requiring both dysfunction and symptoms was considered in the preparation of DSM-5, those charged with this task decided such a change would not be empirically based (see Chapter 3, "Conceptual Framework and Controversies in Adjustment Disorders").

SYMPTOM NUMBER AND DURATION CRITERION

In addition to the distress-impairment criterion, the number and duration of symptoms that are required to make a particular categorical diagnosis are specified in DSM-5 and its predecessors. This information is measured at a cross-section in time, and once the symptom numbers and duration threshold are reached, a diagnostic label is applied provided the distress-impairment criterion (described in the previous section) is also met. For example, the threshold for PTSD is met when 6 of 20 possible symptoms are present for more than 1 month following the type of stressor specified and provided the individual also has clinically significant symptom-related distress or impairment (Box 1–1).

Box 1–1.   DSM-5 Diagnostic Criteria for Posttraumatic Stress Disorder
309.81 (F43.10)

Posttraumatic Stress Disorder

Note: The following criteria apply to adults, adolescents, and children older than 6 years. For children 6 years and younger, see corresponding criteria below.

A. Exposure to actual or threatened death, serious injury, or sexual violence in one (or more) of the following ways:

1. Directly experiencing the traumatic event(s).
2. Witnessing, in person, the event(s) as it occurred to others.
3. Learning that the traumatic event(s) occurred to a close family member or close friend. In cases of actual or threatened death of a family member or friend, the event(s) must have been violent or accidental.
4. Experiencing repeated or extreme exposure to aversive details of the traumatic event(s) (e.g., first responders collecting human remains; police officers repeatedly exposed to details of child abuse).

   Note: Criterion A4 does not apply to exposure through electronic media, television, movies, or pictures, unless this exposure is work-related.

B. Presence of one (or more) of the following intrusion symptoms associated with the traumatic event(s), beginning after the traumatic event(s) occurred:

1. Recurrent, involuntary, and intrusive distressing memories of the traumatic event(s).

   Note: In children older than 6 years, repetitive play may occur in which themes or aspects of the traumatic event(s) are expressed.

2. Recurrent distressing dreams in which the content and/or affect of the dream are related to the traumatic event(s).

   Note: In children, there may be frightening dreams without recognizable content.

3. Dissociative reactions (e.g., flashbacks) in which the individual feels or acts as if the traumatic event(s) were recurring. (Such reactions may occur on a continuum, with the most extreme expression being a complete loss of awareness of present surroundings.)

   Note: In children, trauma-specific reenactment may occur in play.

4. Intense or prolonged psychological distress at exposure to internal or external cues that symbolize or resemble an aspect of the traumatic event(s).

5. Marked physiological reactions to internal or external cues that symbolize or resemble an aspect of the traumatic event(s).

C. Persistent avoidance of stimuli associated with the traumatic event(s), beginning after the traumatic event(s) occurred, as evidenced by one or both of the following:

   1. Avoidance of or efforts to avoid distressing memories, thoughts, or feelings about or closely associated with the traumatic event(s).

   2. Avoidance of or efforts to avoid external reminders (people, places, conversations, activities, objects, situations) that arouse distressing memories, thoughts, or feelings about or closely associated with the traumatic event(s).

D. Negative alterations in cognitions and mood associated with the traumatic event(s), beginning or worsening after the traumatic event(s) occurred, as evidenced by two (or more) of the following:

   1. Inability to remember an important aspect of the traumatic event(s) (typically due to dissociative amnesia and not to other factors such as head injury, alcohol, or drugs).

   2. Persistent and exaggerated negative beliefs or expectations about oneself, others, or the world (e.g., "I am bad," "No one can be trusted," "The world is completely dangerous," "My whole nervous system is permanently ruined").

   3. Persistent, distorted cognitions about the cause or consequences of the traumatic event(s) that lead the individual to blame himself/herself or others.

   4. Persistent negative emotional state (e.g., fear, horror, anger, guilt, or shame).

   5. Markedly diminished interest or participation in significant activities.

   6. Feelings of detachment or estrangement from others.

7. Persistent inability to experience positive emotions (e.g., inability to experience happiness, satisfaction, or loving feelings).

E. Marked alterations in arousal and reactivity associated with the traumatic event(s), beginning or worsening after the traumatic event(s) occurred, as evidenced by two (or more) of the following:

1. Irritable behavior and angry outbursts (with little or no provocation) typically expressed as verbal or physical aggression toward people or objects.
2. Reckless or self-destructive behavior.
3. Hypervigilance.
4. Exaggerated startle response.
5. Problems with concentration.
6. Sleep disturbance (e.g., difficulty falling or staying asleep or restless sleep).

F. Duration of the disturbance (Criteria B, C, D, and E) is more than 1 month.
G. The disturbance causes clinically significant distress or impairment in social, occupational, or other important areas of functioning.
H. The disturbance is not attributable to the physiological effects of a substance (e.g., medication, alcohol) or another medical condition.

Specify whether:

With dissociative symptoms: The individual's symptoms meet the criteria for posttraumatic stress disorder, and in addition, in response to the stressor, the individual experiences persistent or recurrent symptoms of either of the following:

1. **Depersonalization:** Persistent or recurrent experiences of feeling detached from, and as if one were an outside observer of, one's mental processes or body (e.g., feeling as though one were in a dream; feeling a sense of unreality of self or body or of time moving slowly).
2. **Derealization:** Persistent or recurrent experiences of unreality of surroundings (e.g., the world around the individual is experienced as unreal, dreamlike, distant, or distorted).

Note: To use this subtype, the dissociative symptoms must not be attributable to the physiological effects of a substance (e.g., blackouts, behavior during alcohol intoxication) or another medical condition (e.g., complex partial seizures).

Specify if:

With delayed expression: If the full diagnostic criteria are not met until at least 6 months after the event (although the onset and expression of some symptoms may be immediate).

Posttraumatic Stress Disorder for Children 6 Years and Younger

A. In children 6 years and younger, exposure to actual or threatened death, serious injury, or sexual violence in one (or more) of the following ways:

1. Directly experiencing the traumatic event(s).
2. Witnessing, in person, the event(s) as it occurred to others, especially primary caregivers.

Note: Witnessing does not include events that are witnessed only in electronic media, television, movies, or pictures.

3. Learning that the traumatic event(s) occurred to a parent or caregiving figure.

B. Presence of one (or more) of the following intrusion symptoms associated with the traumatic event(s), beginning after the traumatic event(s) occurred:

1. Recurrent, involuntary, and intrusive distressing memories of the traumatic event(s).

   Note: Spontaneous and intrusive memories may not necessarily appear distressing and may be expressed as play reenactment.

2. Recurrent distressing dreams in which the content and/or affect of the dream are related to the traumatic event(s).

   Note: It may not be possible to ascertain that the frightening content is related to the traumatic event.

3. Dissociative reactions (e.g., flashbacks) in which the child feels or acts as if the traumatic event(s) were recurring. (Such reactions may occur on a continuum, with the most extreme expression being a complete loss of awareness of present surroundings.) Such trauma-specific reenactment may occur in play.

4. Intense or prolonged psychological distress at exposure to internal or external cues that symbolize or resemble an aspect of the traumatic event(s).

5. Marked physiological reactions to reminders of the traumatic event(s).

C. One (or more) of the following symptoms, representing either persistent avoidance of stimuli associated with the traumatic event(s) or negative alterations in cognitions and mood associated with the traumatic event(s), must be present, beginning after the event(s) or worsening after the event(s):

Persistent Avoidance of Stimuli

1. Avoidance of or efforts to avoid activities, places, or physical reminders that arouse recollections of the traumatic event(s).

2. Avoidance of or efforts to avoid people, conversations, or interpersonal situations that arouse recollections of the traumatic event(s).

Negative Alterations in Cognitions

3. Substantially increased frequency of negative emotional states (e.g., fear, guilt, sadness, shame, confusion).

4. Markedly diminished interest or participation in significant activities, including constriction of play.

5. Socially withdrawn behavior.

6. Persistent reduction in expression of positive emotions.

D. Alterations in arousal and reactivity associated with the traumatic event(s), beginning or worsening after the traumatic event(s) occurred, as evidenced by two (or more) of the following:

1. Irritable behavior and angry outbursts (with little or no provocation) typically expressed as verbal or physical aggression toward people or objects (including extreme temper tantrums).
2. Hypervigilance.
3. Exaggerated startle response.
4. Problems with concentration.
5. Sleep disturbance (e.g., difficulty falling or staying asleep or restless sleep).

E. The duration of the disturbance is more than 1 month.
F. The disturbance causes clinically significant distress or impairment in relationships with parents, siblings, peers, or other caregivers or with school behavior.
G. The disturbance is not attributable to the physiological effects of a substance (e.g., medication or alcohol) or another medical condition.

Specify whether:

With dissociative symptoms: The individual's symptoms meet the criteria for posttraumatic stress disorder, and the individual experiences persistent or recurrent symptoms of either of the following:

1. **Depersonalization:** Persistent or recurrent experiences of feeling detached from, and as if one were an outside observer of, one's mental processes or body (e.g., feeling as though one were in a dream; feeling a sense of unreality of self or body or of time moving slowly).
2. **Derealization:** Persistent or recurrent experiences of unreality of surroundings (e.g., the world around the individual is experienced as unreal, dreamlike, distant, or distorted).

Note: To use this subtype, the dissociative symptoms must not be attributable to the physiological effects of a substance (e.g., blackouts) or another medical condition (e.g., complex partial seizures).

Specify if:

With delayed expression: If the full diagnostic criteria are not met until at least 6 months after the event (although the onset and expression of some symptoms may be immediate).

Important considerations are how the symptoms for inclusion are selected and how the number and duration thresholds are reached so that individuals without a psychiatric disorder are excluded. These issues are discussed in the following subsections.

Symptoms

Symptoms are derived from those that have been observed and recorded over decades of research into psychiatric conditions. Over time the symptom lists have been altered. As illustrated in Box 1–1, DSM-5 lists 20 symptoms for PTSD and requires a threshold of 6 for diagnosis. However, in DSM-III-R (American Psychiatric Association 1987) and DSM-IV, the total number was 17 with a threshold of 6, although the number required in each cluster of symptoms changed between the two editions. A recent study has shown that using all the possible combinations of symptoms, a total of 636,120 groupings would allow an individual to meet the criteria for PTSD (Galatzer-Levy and Bryant 2013). Thus, far from being a clearly delineated disorder, PTSD as currently defined is very heterogeneous and the symptoms can vary greatly among individuals having the same diagnosis.

This heterogeneity stems from the facts that not all the specified symptoms are required to make the diagnosis and all are regarded as equally important. Therefore, multiple combinations of symptoms are possible. Similarly, in individuals diagnosed with major depression (with the possible exception of the psychotic and melancholic subtypes), the multiplicity of symptoms and their combination result in widely diverse clinical pictures. This is known as the *polythetic approach* to classification. With this approach a diagnosis is made on the basis of a broad set of criteria that are neither necessary nor sufficient. Each member of the category must possess a certain minimal number of defining characteristics, but none of the features has to be found in each member of the category. One way to address this dissimilarity would be to require that certain symptoms are essential to making the diagnosis of PTSD (e.g., flashbacks, reexperiencing the trauma). This would represent the *monothetic approach* in which each category is associated with specific criteria, all of which are considered essential and sufficient to that category's definition (also called *classical categorization*); thus, all the members are identical.

If the polythetic approach is criticized for producing clinical dissimilarities, the monothetic approach is problematic because of the narrowness of the criteria and the possibility of false negatives. A hybrid method could weight some symptoms more than others while not making them sufficient to make a diagnosis.

The PTSD diagnosis has attached weights to four symptom clusters, but these are expressed polythetically (e.g., any one of five intrusion symptoms), so the problem of dissimilarity between those in the diagnostic category continues. A recent study of the distress-impairment criterion in individuals with major depression identified some symptoms (low mood and concentration) as having a significantly greater impact on functioning than others, pointing to the necessity for greater attention to individual symptoms (Fried and Nesse 2014) rather than to overall numbers. In relation to ADs, it has been suggested that if specific symptom criteria are developed, they should be weighted (Baumeister et al. 2009). One symptom mentioned in this regard is affect modulation: this is unimpaired in individuals with ADs in that "the mood state of those with ADs depends more on the cognitive presence of the stressor so that immediate impairment of mood is observed when the stressor is mentioned, while followed by a more pronounced mood recovery when the patient is distracted as compared to those with major depression" (Baumeister et al. 2009, p. 142). It is likely that having fewer symptom criteria and weighting them would greatly reduce the diversity of features in individuals with the same diagnosis.

Duration

An important question regarding duration of mental illness is whether the time thresholds have been derived scientifically or pragmatically. The selection of a particular duration threshold has not received much attention in the trauma- and stressor-related groups of disorders, although in ADs it is recognized that the condition can be prolonged if the stressor or its effects can be prolonged. However, it is not clear why, for example, the latency for the onset of symptoms in ADs is 3 months according to DSM-5 (in ICD-11 it will be 1 month). Also, it is unclear whether the acute stress disorder 1-month cutoff in DSM-5 has been identified scientifically by comparing the predictive power of different time periods associated with the development of PTSD, although it appears not (see Chapter 5, "Acute Stress Disorder").

A similar concern is whether empirical evidence supports the 2-week cutoff for symptoms in major depression. According to Maj (2011), the current cutoff of 2 weeks for major depression has not been validated. Although major depression is not in the trauma- and stressor-related group in DSM-5, it is the most commonly diagnosed condition in psychiatry, and it illustrates the shortcomings of the current classifications.

UTILITY

In deciding on the cutoff between normal and pathological reactions, some argue that diagnosis should be based on the utility that the diagnosis has for the doctor and the patient. An example suggested by First (2011) is that a cost-benefit analysis of providing mood disorder treatment at a particular threshold could be compared with the impact on various outcome measures of using a different threshold. Maj (2011) also suggests that thresholds could vary depending on the purpose. He suggests that in major depression the threshold for a condition to warrant psychiatric attention should be lower than that for initiating pharmacotherapy. The suggestion that the threshold for psychiatric input and various interventions is variable also applies to ADs, for which a referral for the purpose of observation would occur at a lower threshold than would the initiation of a treatment such as cognitive therapy.

SUBTHRESHOLD DISORDERS

If the distress-impairment or threshold (symptom number and duration) criteria are not met, then the diagnosis cannot be made. Arguably, this situation should lead to the assumption that no disorder is present; however, the profession continues to have an interest in individuals who are symptomatic, even when they do not meet the criteria for a full-blown disorder. These persons are said to have subthreshold disorders. The rationale for paying attention to subthreshold conditions is that they may be associated with functional impairment, and therefore individuals should receive treatment for subthreshold PTSD (Zlotnick et al. 2002) and for subthreshold depressive disorders (Ayuso-Mateos et al. 2010). There are several reasons why the symptom threshold for a particular disorder may not be reached in an individual. First, the person may have only partially responded to or is in the process of responding to an intervention for a prior disorder and is exhibiting residual symptoms at the time of interview. Second, the symptoms may represent a condition in evolution that has not yet solidified into a recognized syndrome. Third, the person is experiencing the normal vagaries of life that produce understandable emotional reactions, easily conflated with psychiatric disorders as discussed earlier (see "Symptom Number and Duration Criterion"). In these situations there is good reason to simply watch and wait rather than embarking on a particular intervention at that point.

The recommendation that subthreshold conditions require treatment bolsters the charge that the construct of subthreshold disorders amounts to the overreach of psychiatry into ordinary distress. As an unintended consequence, the profession could stand accused of causing potential harm by prescribing either medication or psychotherapy when there may not be any clinical indication to do so and side effects result. The inclusion of individuals not meeting criteria for the various syndromes as being in need of treatment could also lead to huge inflation in prevalence estimates (Frances 2009). This practice undermines the immediate purpose of classification, which is to separate those who are ill from those who are not. However, there also is merit in monitoring individuals who have ongoing symptoms at a subthreshold level to exclude the possibility of an emergent disorder. These issues are considered in further detail in Chapter 3 with respect to ADs.

THE DIMENSIONAL APPROACH

In light of the absence of clear demarcations between different psychiatric disorders and between normality and mental illness, some authors have proposed the use of dimensional measures instead of categorical labels (Frances 2009; Kendell and Jablensky 2003) or, alternatively, a combination of both to augment each other. The dimensions might include biological measures, symptom severity scores, or measures of social functioning, although little work has been done on them. Despite all the problems with the categorical approach, however, there is no agreement on which dimensions should be measured or to which diagnostic groups they should apply. Discussions on applying a dimensional model to the personality disorder groups have a long history, although categories are still included in DSM-5. A further concern with dimensions is what effect this approach would have on doctor-patient and doctor-doctor communication or on research. Importantly, a dimensional approach would not assist in deciding on the boundary between what is a normal reaction to stress and what is pathological unless the cutoff point was defined by research evidence.

In an attempt to capture the continuum from normality to pathology that is the hallmark of mental illness, DSM-5 has incorporated a dimensional as well as categorical approach. This allows the gradient in domains, which is obscured by a simple categorical approach, to be captured. The process involves three stages (see DSM-5 "Assessment Measures," pp. 733–737). The first stage involves administration of the Level 1 Cross-Cutting Symptom Measure. The adult version measures 13 core domains (e.g., depression, anger, psychosis, personality functioning) using 23 self-rated questions. The second stage is initiated if an individual scores at least 2 (mild) out of 5 on any item in a domain. The Level 2 Cross-Cutting Symptom Measures provide more detailed information on the symptoms within that domain. For example, individuals scoring at least 2 in the Level 1 depression domain would be administered the Patient Reported Outcomes Measurement Information System (PROMIS) Emotional Distress–Depression—Short Form at Level 2 (available online at www.psychiatry.org/practice/dsm/dsm5/online-assessment-measures#Level2), and this could be used to establish the severity of symptoms and track them over time. The third stage involves a clinical assessment to make a diagnosis. The DSM-5 Web site also includes the World Health Organization Disability Assessment Schedule (WHODAS), which can be used to track changes in overall functioning as clinically indicated. Clearly, these assessments are intricate.

Notwithstanding the attempts to introduce dimensional measures into DSM-5, it is questionable whether these measures will be used because the dimensional measures that were incorporated into DSM-IV, such as measures of severity and the 100-point Global Assessment of Functioning Scale, were seldom used either in practice or in research (Frances 2009), possibly because they were regarded as burdensome. Frances (2009) commented that dimensions are "appealing ideas whose time has not yet arrived" (p. 391). It is also unlikely that the combined use of dimensions and categories will assist in separating normal responses to stress from pathological responses.

CLINICAL JUDGMENT

The original idea behind DSM-III was to improve the reliability of psychiatric diagnosis, which had been a source of great difficulty because it relied heavily on the vagaries of clinical judgment. In deciding on the line between normal and pathological, developers of DSM have attempted to deal with this by using the clinical significance (symptoms or impairment) and threshold criteria. However, many commentators question this approach (Horwitz and Wakefield 2007).

DSM-III, DSM-IV, and DSM-5 all place an emphasis on clinical judgment alongside the application of specific criteria. However, some authors have expressed concern that diagnosis has largely become a cursory exercise, divorced from the thorough clinical assessment and reflective approach recommended by these manuals (McHugh and Slavney 2012). They argue that the bottom-up approach, in which detailed information is gleaned from the patient, third parties, and an evaluation of the person's life history, has been replaced by a top-down approach, in which diagnosis is based on symptom checklists. A World Health Organization survey of international psychiatrists found that the majority wanted diagnostic manuals to contain flexible guidance rather than fixed diagnostic criteria so that clinical judgment could be factored into diagnostic decision making (Reed et al. 2011). Additionally, some authors have called for clinicians to make the decision as to whether a response to a stressor was proportionate or excessive (Horwitz and Wakefield 2007), whereas others have seen this as "more a step backward than forward for our field," pointing to the subjectivity of deciding on "understandability" (Kendler 2008, p. 150). These issues are illustrated in the vignette below.

Case Vignette

Mr. X claimed to have been adversely affected by problems in his workplace, where he worked in middle management in information technology. He claimed to have been bullied by his manager and gave examples of being verbally humiliated and shouted at in front of his peers. He said he experienced initial insomnia, psychic symptoms of anxiety but no physical symptoms, impaired concentration, and irritability at how he was being treated. He continued to work, although he found it difficult and dreaded going to work each day. His mood was low, and he had to have time off every few weeks. He worried constantly about his problems at work. His general practitioner prescribed a selective serotonin reuptake inhibitor as an antidepressant, but the medication had no effect on his work-related symptoms. However, Mr. X enjoyed the company of his family, playing golf with friends, and going on family trips, during which his symptoms dissipated.

The clinician was asked to provide a report by Mr. X's attorney because Mr. X was claiming psychological injury. The patient could have been diagnosed with an AD because the symptoms arose in a particular context and disappeared when he was away from the source of his problems or with major depression because he reached the distress-impairment criterion and the symptom duration threshold if one adhered rigidly to DSM-5. The diagnosis made was of an adjustment disorder because Mr. X had both symptoms and dysfunction requiring time off work. Mr. X obtained a severance package from work and his symptoms resolved. Two months later he found new employment.

This vignette illustrates the problem of ignoring the primacy that clinical judgment would likely accord the context of the symptoms and instead basing diagnosis on symptom thresholds.

Stimulated by the controversy that removal of the bereavement exclusion generated and by concerns about the overdiagnosis of psychiatric disorders, DSM-5 makes reference to clinical judgment in deciding how to distinguish illness from normality in the context of bereavement. A note accompanying the diagnostic criteria for major depression tentatively suggests the following:

> Although such symptoms may be understandable or considered appropriate to the loss, the presence of a major depressive episode in addition to the normal response to a significant loss should also be carefully considered. This decision inevitably requires the exercise of clinical judgment based on the individual's history and the cultural norms for the expression of distress in the context of loss. (American Psychiatric Association 2013, p. 161)

Although this description might be seen as ambivalent, a lengthy footnote goes on to assist the clinician by outlining in significant detail the likely differences in the expression of dysphoria in normal grief, in thought content, in self-esteem, and in other aspects of grief (American Psychiatric Association 2013, p. 161). More generally, DSM-5 is positive about clinical judgment, although it falls short of using of that phrase:

> [I]t is not sufficient to simply check off the symptoms in the diagnostic criteria to make a mental disorder diagnosis…. It requires clinical training to recognize when the combination of predisposing, precipitating, perpetuating, and protective factors has resulted in a psychopathological condition in which physical signs and symptoms exceed normal ranges. (American Psychiatric Association 2013, p. 19)

Notwithstanding the development of describing the features of normal grief and of according weight to clinical judgment, some researchers (e.g., Maj 2013) believe it is unclear whether the clinician has complete freedom in these circumstances or whether a diagnosis of major depression is compelled once the criteria are met even if culturally the features seem to represent a normal grief response. This uncertainty could lead to *interpretation bias,* or the tendency to falsely interpret the meaning of the guidance provided. At least the approach of DSM-5 in the bereavement exclusion–major depression controversy is a nod in the direction of the exercise of clinical judgment. No such guidance is given regarding the reactions to other stressors, such as the breakup of a relationship, the loss of a beloved pet, the onset of a potentially life-threatening illness, and so on, and this is a consideration for future modifications of DSM-5.

CONCLUSION

DSM-5 places much emphasis on clinical judgment. The fact that judgment plays such a major role in determining what is normal and what is excessive in response to psychosocial stressors places a huge onus on the clinician. In the absence of biological markers to demarcate the boundaries between various disorders, clinicians are left with only clinical judgment.

Three avenues of research might enhance clinical judgment. The first is for research to turn its attention to symptom weighting so that clinicians can judge the importance of certain symptoms when compared with others in relation to the individual patient rather than assuming that each symptom carries equal weight. The second is use of a monothetic approach to delineate homogeneous groups with identical symptoms. The third avenue is to reopen the study of clinical judgment itself and of the diagnostic process. Clinimetrics is "a domain concerned with the measurement of clinical issues that do not find room in customary clinical taxonomy" (Fava et al. 2014, p. 137), and it embraces a range of elements such as the types, severity patterns, and sequencing of symptoms as well as illness progression. Context and culture could also be taken into account because these are elements that are frequently captured by clinical judgment and that the clinician brings to bear in making diagnostic and treatment decisions. Perhaps the time has arrived for clinimetrics.

DSM-5 and its predecessors have many imperfections, but they have enabled a rich research base with which to move into the future. Although problems of reliability are much less prominent, time will tell if the goal of achieving validity for the syndromes that are recognized will also be achieved.

Key Points

- For the most part there are no clear-cut demarcations between normal and pathological reactions to stress based on symptoms.

- The hope that psychobiological measures distinguishing some disorders would assist in the development of DSM-5 has not been realized.

- Attempts to differentiate pathological from normal reactions have focused on the presence of impairment or distress and on duration and symptom number thresholds. Impairment and distress are problematic because they cannot be operationalized and are likely to result in overdiagnosis (false positives) and in widely different clinical pictures for individuals with the same diagnosis, stemming from the polythetic approach to classification.

- One approach to improving diagnostic validity would be to have symptom weightings and move toward a monothetic or mixed approach.

- Individuals with symptoms that fall short of the threshold criterion are often classified as having subthreshold conditions, which can also potentially lead to overtreatment.

- In DSM-5, dimensional measures have been combined with categorical diagnosis in an attempt to deal with the continuum from normality to psychopathology, but it is unclear whether these dimensional measures will be used by clinicians.

- Clinical judgment remains central to diagnosis, and this is clearly recognized in DSM-5, although this centrality, too, has its critics.

- Efforts to provide clinicians with clear guidance on the features of normal and pathological reactions to stress should continue, and the process of clinical diagnosis is worthy of research.

SUGGESTED READINGS

Kendall R: The Role of Diagnosis in Psychiatry, New York, Blackwell Science, 1975 (Although this book is old, limited copies are still available. It addresses issues such as the purpose of diagnosis, validity, dimensions, and zones of rarity in a very accessible style.)

Stein D, Lund C, Nesse RM: Classification systems in psychiatry: diagnosis and global mental health in an era of DSM-5 and ICD-11. Curr Opin Psychiatry 26(5):493–497, 2013

REFERENCES

American Psychiatric Association: Diagnostic and Statistical Manual of Mental Disorders, 3rd Edition. Washington, DC, American Psychiatric Association, 1980

American Psychiatric Association: Diagnostic and Statistical Manual of Mental Disorders, 3rd Edition, Revised. Washington, DC, American Psychiatric Association, 1987

American Psychiatric Association: Diagnostic and Statistical Manual of Mental Disorders, 4th Edition. Washington, DC, American Psychiatric Association, 1994

American Psychiatric Association: Diagnostic and Statistical Manual of Mental Disorders, 5th Edition. Arlington, VA, American Psychiatric Association, 2013

Ayuso-Mateos JL, Nuevo R, Verdes E, et al: From depressive symptoms to depressive disorders: the relevance of thresholds. Br J Psychiatry 196(5):365–371, 2010 20435961

Baumeister H, Maercker A, Casey P: Adjustment disorder with depressed mood: a critique of its DSM-IV and ICD-10 conceptualisations and recommendations for the future. Psychopathology 42(3):139–147, 2009 19276640

Casey P, Birbeck G, McDonagh C, et al: Personality disorder, depression and functioning: results from the ODIN study. J Affect Disord 82(2):277–283, 2004 15488258

Casey P, Maracy M, Kelly BD, et al: Can adjustment disorder and depressive episode be distinguished? Results from ODIN. J Affect Disord 92(2–3):291–297, 2006 16515807

Clarke DM, Kissane DW: Demoralization: its phenomenology and importance. Aust NZ J Psychiatry 36(6):733–742, 2002 12406115

Cooper R: Avoiding false positives: zones of rarity, the threshold problem and the DSM clinical significance criterion. Can J Psychiatry 58(11):606–611, 2013 24246430

Fava GA, Guidi J, Grandi S, et al: The missing link between clinical states and biomarkers in mental disorders. Psychother Psychosom 83(3):136–141, 2014 24732705

First MB: DSM-5 proposals for mood disorders: a cost-benefit analysis. Curr Opin Psychiatry 24(1):1–9, 2011 21042219

Frances A: Problems in defining clinical significance in epidemiological studies. Arch Gen Psychiatry 55(2):119, 1998 9477923

Frances A: Whither DSM-V? Br J Psychiatry 195(5):391–392, 2009 19880926

Fried EI, Nesse RM: The impact of individual depressive symptoms on impairment of psychosocial functioning. PLoS One 9(2):e90311, 2014 24587318

Galatzer-Levy IR Bryant RA: 636,120 ways to have posttraumatic stress disorder. Perspect Psychol Sci 8(6):651–662, 2013

Healy D: Dysphoria, in Symptoms of Depression. Edited by Costello CG. New York, Wiley, 1993, pp 24–25

Helmchen H, Linden M: Subthreshold disorders in psychiatry: clinical reality, methodological artifact, and the double-threshold problem. Compr Psychiatry 41(2 suppl 1):1–7, 2000 10746897

Horwitz M, Wakefield JC: The Loss of Sadness: How Psychiatry Transformed Normal Sorrow Into Depressive Disorder. Oxford, UK, Oxford University Press, 2007

Jaspers K: Allgemeine psychopathologie (1913), in General Psychopathology, Volumes 1 and 2. Translated by Hoenig J, Hamilton MW. Baltimore, MD, Johns Hopkins University Press, 1997, pp 1–992

Kendell R, Jablensky A: Distinguishing between the validity and utility of psychiatric diagnoses. Am J Psychiatry 160(1):4–12, 2003 12505793

Kendler K: Book review. The Loss of Sadness: How Psychiatry Transformed Normal Sorrow Into Depressive Disorder, by Horwitz AV and Wakefield JC. Psychol Med 38:148–150, 2008

Maj M: When does depression become a mental disorder? Br J Psychiatry 199(2):85–86, 2011

Maj M: From "madness" to "mental health problems": reflections on the evolving target of psychiatry. World Psychiatry 11(3):137–138, 2012 23024663

Maj M: "Clinical judgment" and the DSM-5 diagnosis of major depression. World Psychiatry 12(2):89–91, 2013 23737407

Mapother E: Manic-depressive psychosis. Br Med J 2:872–877, 1926

McHugh PR, Slavney PR: Mental illness—comprehensive evaluation or checklist? N Engl J Med 366(20):1853–1855, 2012 22591291

Narrow WE, Rae DS, Robins LN, et al: Revised prevalence estimates of mental disorders in the United States: using a clinical significance criterion to reconcile 2 surveys' estimates. Arch Gen Psychiatry 59(2):115–123, 2002 11825131

Parker G: Is major depression that major? Acta Psychiatr Scand 129(6):458–459, 2014 23952660

Reed GM, Mendonça Correia J, Esparza P, et al: The WPA-WHO global survey of psychiatrists' attitudes towards mental disorders classification. World Psychiatry 10(2):118–131, 2011 21633689

Reynolds M, Brewin CR: Intrusive memories in depression and posttraumatic stress disorder. Behav Res Ther 37(3):201–215, 1999 10087639

Spitzer R: The diagnostic status of homosexuality in DSM-III: a reformulation of the issues. Am J Psychiatry 138(2):210–215, 1981 7457641

Stein DJ, Phillips KA, Bolton D, et al: What is a mental/psychiatric disorder? From DSM-IV to DSM-V. Psychol Med 40(11):1759–1765, 2010 20624327

Stein DJ, Lund C, Nesse RM: Classification systems in psychiatry: diagnosis and global mental health in an era of DSM-5 and ICD-11. Curr Opin Psychiatry 26(5):493–497, 2013 23867662

Wakefield J: Diagnosing DSM-IV—part 1: DSM-IV and the concept of disorder. Behav Res Ther 35(7):633–649, 1997

World Health Organization: International Statistical Classification of Diseases and Related Health Problems, 10th Revision. Geneva, World Health Organization, 1992

Zlotnick C, Franklin CL, Zimmerman M: Does "subthreshold" posttraumatic stress disorder have any clinical relevance? Compr Psychiatry 43(6):413–419, 2002 12439826

Limits to the Phenomenological Approach to the Diagnosis of Adjustment Disorders

Peter Tyrer, M.D.

HISTORY OF PHENOMENOLOGY

As pointed out in Chapter 1, "Borderline Between Normal and Pathological Responses," Karl Jaspers is the father of phenomenology in psychiatry, and it was he who, almost single-handedly, developed phenomenology as a scientific subject to buttress, and often replace, the somewhat unsatisfactory description of psychopathology (mainly derived from psychodynamic theory) being used early in the twentieth century. In his seminal textbook, *General Psychopathology* (Jaspers 1913/1997), he referred to a set of "psychological reactions," which could themselves become disorders. He called these *reactive disorders,* defined as those conditions that had a clear connection to a precipitating event. This adumbrated the field of stress and adjustment disorders (ADs) that has persisted in all classifications to this day.

The major problem with these disorders in phenomenology is the presence of two separate elements: 1) the manifestations of the disorder in terms of symptoms, behavior, and expression and 2) the causes defined in terms of environmental precipitants. These two elements often clash. For example, a study on the epidemiology of posttraumatic stress disorder (PTSD) showed that most people who satisfied the phenomenological and diagnostic requirements of PTSD did not have a serious precipitating traumatic event (Mol et al. 2005). The main results of this study are shown in Table 2–1.

Although there was a clear accepted traumatic event preceding the onset of symptoms satisfying the diagnosis of PTSD in 284 cases, there were nearly twice as many cases (519) in which exactly the same criteria in terms of phenomenology followed events that were not, according to the diagnostic system, regarded as traumatic. The most common of these was the death of a close relative. Moreover, the study also found that in general, the key symptoms of PTSD—reexperiencing, avoidance, and arousal—were more prominent following nontraumatic events than traumatic ones. These findings expose the risks of yoking together etiology and phenomenology in diagnosis.

PHENOMENOLOGY, DSM, AND RELIABILITY

It is a matter of argument whether phenomenology is a science. Science depends on measurement and independent validation, and phenomenology of mental illness constitutes a formal description of the subjective experiences of psychiatric patients without any independent confirmation that they are true. The subjective experiences of a patient with delirium associated with physical illness and those of a patient with schizophrenia can be remarkably similar, although the causes are very different. However, phenomenology is not valueless. If there is no good way of communicating the experiences of patients to others, every single psychiatric phenomenon becomes a unique event that will never again be experienced in the same way. The advantage of phenomenology is that it groups the common elements of psychiatric disorders in a meaningful way. The meaning may not necessarily be a manifestation of truth, but it represents a practical way of communicating between professionals and also aids to some extent in diagnosis.

Psychiatric classifications rely on a mix of hard objective data (e.g., a magnetic resonance imaging scan), softer objective data (e.g., neuropsychological testing), and careful clinical observation (observed behavior, symptoms, and phenomenology). Before DSM-III was published (American Psychiatric Association 1980), these classifications were in disarray; although consistency of diagnosis could be achieved within an individual over the course of time, tremendous inconsistency existed among psychiatrists in their interpretation of mental manifestations of illness.

As recently as the early 1970s, there was a considerable divergence of opinion between American and British psychiatrists about the diagnosis of schizo-

TABLE 2–1.   Comparison of posttraumatic stress disorder profiles of patients after traumatic and life events

	n^a	Total log PTSD score[b] (mean)	Original score (geometric mean)
Traumatic events			
Accidents	42	0.53	2.4
Sudden death of loved one (not murder or unknown whether murder)	142	0.58	2.8
Witnessing violence	4	0.60	3.0
Disaster	16	0.61	3.1
Murder or suicide of loved one	26	0.68	3.8
War	23	0.71	4.1
Robbery	5	0.88	6.6
Physical abuse (adult)	9	0.94	7.7
Sexual abuse (adult)	4	1.09	11.3
Physical abuse or sexual abuse (child)	13	1.09	11.3
Life events			
Burglary without confrontation of burglar	11	0.54	2.5
Death of loved one (nonsudden or unclear whether sudden or not)	208	0.59	2.9
Miscellaneous, not traumatic	14	0.61	3.1
(Chronic) illness of loved one	95	0.71	4.1
Serious illness (self)	91	0.82	5.6
Problems with study/work	19	0.83	5.8
Relational problems	81	0.88	6.6

Note.   PTSD = posttraumatic stress disorder.
[a]Data missing in 29 cases.
[b]Score is $\log_{10}$ (PTSD score + 1).
Source.   Reprinted from Mol et al. 2005. Available at http://bjp.rcpsych.org/content/186/6/494. Used with permission.

phrenia. In the U.S.-U.K. Diagnostic Project (Cooper et al. 1972; Sharpe et al. 1974), clinicians in both countries assessed vignettes of psychiatric patients and came to a set of poor agreement levels; the agreement was worst for the diagnosis of schizophrenia. Work at the Washington University School of Medicine, under the far-seeing Samuel Guze, was also a major influence, helping to remove the notion that somatic symptoms were equivalent to conversion symptoms (Guze et al. 1971), defining the importance of follow-up studies (Guze 1970; Guze et al. 1986), and setting forth the notion that diagnosis might be best made by clearly defined operational criteria (Feighner et al. 1972).

Forty years later, the self-confidence of these pioneers has been replaced by a heavy aura of doubt among psychiatrists. Successive DSM revisions have received greater criticism than their predecessors, and the absence of any independent validation has troubled those responsible for reforming classification systems. David Kupfer, chair of the DSM-5 Task Force, wrote gloomily at the beginning of their deliberations that it was disturbing that

> not one laboratory marker has been found to be specific in identifying any of the DSM-defined syndromes. Epidemiologic and clinical studies have shown extremely high rates of comorbidity among the disorders, undermining the hypothesis that the syndromes represent distinct etiologies. Furthermore, epidemiologic studies have shown a high degree of short-term diagnostic instability for many disorders. With regard to treatment, lack of treatment specificity is the rule rather than the exception. (Kupfer 2002, p. xvii)

Many people are now becoming disillusioned with the DSM classification because it gives a spurious impression of solidity in diagnostic practice that is lacking for many of the disorders (e.g., Paris 2013). The considered view that diagnosis is still developing but is overall going forward has been expressed by Craddock and Mynors-Wallis (2014):

> The future is likely to require a willingness to use both categorical and dimensional approaches. It will also be necessary to ensure consistency between the diagnoses used in all aspects of medicine that relate to brain and behavioral disorders. Further, like all medical classifications, it is likely to involve a pragmatic mix of approaches that reflect the differing levels of understanding of each diagnostic entity. (p. 94)

Few would disagree that some form of classification is essential for effective communication with colleagues and with the general public and that if every problem is considered unique, there is little to be gained from previous knowledge. The success of DSM-III was largely grounded on the evidence that it was possible for psychiatrists to agree on diagnostic categories at a sufficiently acceptable level and to scotch the medical student joke that "a psychiatrist is a doctor who disagrees with his colleagues." Put simply, a good DSM-III diagnosis made sense across the board.

There was no need to write reams of qualifying information to communicate the essential nature of the condition, and therefore DSM-III was a great step forward.

What has been realized in the ensuing years is that good reliability is not enough to make a good diagnosis. Trained assessors can always achieve good reliability, but a highly reliable diagnosis can still be completely invalid. For example, members of the Flat Earth Society have been trained, at least in one sense, to believe that the Earth is flat, and therefore the reliability of the operational criterion "the Earth is flat" would achieve a correlation of 1.0, but only for this trained group. As a consequence of this realization about reliability and diagnosis, the emphasis on operational criteria as the gold standard of diagnosis has suffered a serious knock, and subsequent editions of DSM, despite accommodating this concern, have been viewed much more circumspectly and often critically, especially when they seem to have expanded to include what many would consider to be normal variation that is not pathological (Frances 2013).

SPECIAL PROBLEMS WITH THE DIAGNOSIS OF ADJUSTMENT DISORDERS

Stress and ADs differ from all other mental state disorders because of the relevance of three components: etiology, phenomenology, and time. Several other diagnostic groups rely on two of these, but this is the only group that requires consideration of all three. This has led to particular problems in diagnosis because when there is discordance across the three components, some puzzlement is created and a clinician often has to make arbitrary decisions. It is useful to discuss the implications of the combinations of these three elements.

Etiology, Phenomenology, and Time Are All Concordant

In a classical account of an AD, the patient is normally well adjusted and has little or no evidence of psychiatric disorder before the onset of the adjustment reaction. He or she then experiences a significant degree of traumatic or nontraumatic stress and develops symptoms, most commonly of anxiety and depression, but these are not sufficient to reach the status of the DSM disorder. These symptoms are clearly related to the stress to which the person has been exposed, and the expectation is that in the absence of continuing stress there will be a relatively rapid resolution of the problem.

In this case there is no real dispute over the diagnosis of an AD. There is no other place in the DSM classification for such a condition, and although the condition is likely to be self-limiting, there is still an important degree of distress that needs to be acknowledged by the clinician.

Etiology and Phenomenology Are Concordant but Time Is Not

It is not uncommon for symptoms of an AD to persist for very many months. This is because the nature of the stress also becomes persistent. For example, people living in a chronic war zone or a partner in a marriage in which there is continuous conflict can experience the symptoms of an AD over a long period precisely because the stress has not gone away. The major difficulty in such a case is that continuous symptoms, even if relatively mild, can cross the threshold for a DSM disorder such as major depression. Nonetheless, if it is absolutely clear that the stress is a major precipitant of the symptomatology, most clinicians would not have difficulty in describing the condition as primarily an AD.

Etiology and Time Are Concordant but Phenomenology Is Not

In the DSM-5 classification of ADs (American Psychiatric Association 2013), there is still the requirement in the diagnosis to specify the subtype, characterized by depressed mood, anxious symptoms, and/or disturbances in conduct. However, it is quite possible for patients to experience a wide range of symptoms in response to stress, and this is recognized in the original DSM-III criteria for AD. The purist might well ask, "Where is the evidence that depressive and anxiety symptoms and conduct problems are the only consequences of the type of stress that occurs in ADs?" If an individual displays marked obsessional checking behavior leading to significant distress as a direct consequence of a family member's becoming ill, does this not also qualify as an AD if the level of symptoms is lower than that required for the diagnosis of obsessive-compulsive disorder?

The clinician is then placed in a dilemma. The patient seems to satisfy all the criteria for an AD, but the phenomenology does not fit in with one of the specified categories of symptomatology or behavior. My expectation is that the average clinician in such a situation would still diagnose the condition as an AD but select *unspecified* for the subtype. It could be argued that a category "other symptoms and behavior" would be equally appropriate in the diagnostic criteria.

A much more common example of phenomenology being discordant in the case of ADs is when there is a clear relationship between the symptomatology and external (or internal) stress but the nature of the symptomatology crosses the threshold to a formal DSM-5 disorder. This is a much more difficult predicament for the clinician. In a study that has influenced my practice, patients with DSM-III anxiety and depressive disorders often experienced remission of their symptoms in a very short time after beginning treatment, often too short a time to lead to the conclusion that the improvement was due to a direct treatment response. More significantly, 5 years later these patients tended to remain well and were significantly more improved than those patients who still had significant symptoms at 6 weeks of treatment (Seivewright et al. 1998; Tyrer et al. 2004). The researchers concluded that it probably would have been better to diagnose many of these people as having ADs, not least because once this diagnosis is made it is often unnecessary to embark on complex, potentially long-term treatments. Put another way, if DSM diagnoses are made purely on the basis of symptomatology and phenomenology, then a large number of self-limiting conditions will be treated unnecessarily, with the consequent dangers of iatrogenesis. This is illustrated in the following case example.

Case Vignette

Mrs. E, age 65 years, was brought to an outpatient clinic by her daughter. She was in a state of great distress because 2 weeks earlier she was told that her son, age 40, had been killed in a car accident 250 miles away. She could not stop thinking about his death and blamed herself for not having arranged for him to get new tires on his car when he last stayed with her. She was examined by a psychiatrist-in-training, who came into the consultant's office later to describe his findings: "This patient has classical severe depressive illness with some symptoms of PTSD," he stated confidently. "She cannot sleep for more than a few hours, keeps waking in the night, will hardly eat anything, and cannot face each new day. She is excessively anxious and aroused and keeps going over the accident in her own mind. She became very distressed when coming with her daughter in the car today because she was very afraid of what might happen and could not stop thinking about her son." After some further comments he concluded, "I think she needs to be prescribed antidepressants, and we should be thinking of referring her for psychological therapy, probably trauma-focused cognitive-behavioral therapy."

The consultant decided to see Mrs. E and her daughter. Both were now a great deal calmer, and he elicited some additional information from them both. Mrs. E had not had any mental illness previously, had always coped with adversity well in the past, and 2 years previously had nursed her husband at home until his death after he was diagnosed with pancreatic cancer. She was rather scornful of people with mental illness and had the old-fashioned view that people should learn how to cope with adversity without seeking outside help.

The consultant came to the view that Mrs. E's problem was best formulated as an AD in spite of the undoubted presence of both depressive and PTSD symptoms. After discussion with both Mrs. E and her daughter, the consultant decided to prescribe only a nighttime sedative, to be taken as needed, and asked Mrs. E to return in 2 weeks after her son's funeral. At the time of the follow-up appointment, she was still somewhat distressed but was pleased she had been to the funeral and "kept myself together," and she was sleeping better. At an appointment 3 months later, she was noted to be very well and was discharged.

In evaluating this case it is easy to see how formal diagnosis can get in the way of good practice. The junior doctor has been well trained; he understands the diagnostic guidelines of both major depressive disorder and PTSD, and there seems little doubt that the patient is close to satisfying the requirements for both diagnoses, although some practitioners might be cautious because the time frame of symptoms is quite short. He clearly feels something needs to be done in the way of active treatment. Mrs. E is a patient in deep distress and with the potential of developing much greater pathology. She may also be considered to be at risk of suicide. The phenomenology of the disorder is also unequivocal; Mrs. E is reexperiencing symptoms, showing signs of avoidance, and is highly aroused. She also has poor appetite, severe sleep disturbance, and depressed mood.

So why did the consultant not follow the trainee's suggestion? The answer is because the consultant used clinical judgment based on the additional information he had found at his separate interview. The exercise of clinical judgment is the elephant in the room of diagnosis. It cannot be defined or quantified in the way that nosologists would like it to be and therefore is generally ignored in the formal diagnostic process, but it is nonetheless essential to good practice and is recognized as being of prime importance in the process of assessment (McHugh and Slavney 2012). It even enters into the DSM diagnostic process, as noted in Chapter 1. Clinical judgment in the case of Mrs. E led to some very important consequences that were based on the following information:

1. Mrs. E had never had any psychiatric disorder before this present episode.
2. She had been successful before in coping with adversity.
3. She did not take kindly to pathologizing mental distress.

This information led to the opinion, guess, or judgment (whichever is preferred) that Mrs. E had sufficient internal resources to be able to overcome the stress of her son's death with a minimum of outside help. The role of personality is highly relevant when diagnosing an AD. When an individual such as Mrs. E has reached an advanced age without experiencing any psychiatric illness and has coped with previous adversity well, then it is reasonable to suppose that her powers of resilience are better than average. It is therefore not surprising that the consultant judged that despite the intensity of Mrs. E's current symptoms, specific therapy for her depression and stress disorder was not needed. In these circumstances phenomenology is ignored, and rightly so. The architects of recent DSM classifications have recognized this problem and advised clinicians to be wary of diagnosing ADs in the presence of personality disorders. In fact, ADs should be more commonly diagnosed in the presence of personality strengths, and when personality weaknesses are more prominent, the diagnoses of PTSD and depressive episode are more likely to be appropriate (Doherty et al. 2014).

Summary

What is clear from examination of these three different elements of ADs—etiology, phenomenology, and time—is that the exact nature of the phenomenology is of relatively little weight, if any at all, in determining the diagnosis. All too often it seems to get in the way rather than to aid the diagnosis. To some extent this has been acknowledged in the new criteria for DSM-5, because when using DSM-IV criteria (American Psychiatric Association 1994), clinicians tended to diagnose an AD for any patient with a hodgepodge of residual symptomatology that did not satisfy any particular diagnosis.

IMPACT OF RESEARCH DIAGNOSTIC CRITERIA ON DIAGNOSIS OF ADJUSTMENT DISORDERS

The National Institute of Mental Health (NIMH) in the United States is at the forefront of research development. Therefore, when the NIMH makes pungent criticisms of both DSM and ICD and formulates a radically different model of classification of mental disorders, a great deal of debate and rethinking is likely to follow. The Research Domain Criteria (RDoC) model, proposed by Thomas Insel (2014) of NIMH and his colleagues, uses, probably correctly, the overused phrase "paradigm shift" in reviewing the classification of mental disorders. This model does not accept the traditional view of mental disorders as symptom complexes that can be identified through clinical description. Instead, it examines the primary behavioral functions of the brain and the neural systems that are responsible for implementing this behavior. Because RDoC is a biobehavioral model, it might be thought that it would be so far removed from ADs—perhaps the most classical diagnosis emphasizing the importance of social psychiatry— that it would have little to offer.

However, this is not the case. Cuthbert and Insel (2013) recently reformulated the seven pillars of RDoC, which are summarized in Table 2–2. What is immediately clear from these central elements is that the diagnosis of ADs would benefit overall from the adoption of this domain approach. The word *domain* is an appropriate one here because it describes the territory of disorder. Rather than walling off specific areas for diagnostic purposes, it asks the clinician to look at the whole area covered by the symptoms or behavior. The same general principle has been used in the ICD-11 revised classification of personality disorder (Tyrer et al. 2015). Even though the link between neural mechanisms and behavior in most psychiatric disorders is a long way off, it would help greatly if ADs received at least as much attention as the much more extensively studied PTSD.

The arguments about the number of symptom groups necessary for the diagnosis of PTSD, which show no signs of abating (Forbes et al. 2015; O'Donnell et al. 2014), will not lead to a significant step forward for science. They may help clinicians a little, but without a better guiding principle they can only end as a soggy consensus, ready to be overturned by the next diagnostic algorithm.

TABLE 2–2.   Implications of the Research Domain Criteria (RDoC) for the study of adjustment disorders

Seven pillars of RDoC	Central elements	Relevance to adjustment disorders
Translational research perspective	Basic science in the driving force behind the classification	Of some relevance because there is abundant evidence of neurobiological and behavioral consequences of stress
Dimensional approach to classification	Need to accommodate the full range of normality and pathology	Adjustment disorders are a good exemplar of a condition that has been neglected as outside the range of mainstream psychopathology but that is highly relevant to personal distress and functioning
Development of reliable and valid measures of diagnosis	Need for measures that are not artificially diagnosis-specific and that cover the range of all pathology	Highly relevant in adjustment disorders. The so-called stress disorders need to be accommodated as a broad group with standard measurements for all
Broader design of research studies	Need to acknowledge that treatments are effective across a range of disorders and the important variables are rarely diagnostic ones	Acceptance that adjustment disorders should be studied together with other stress disorders, not regarded as a separate entity
Integration of behavior and neural science	Importance of fact that neural science determines behavior	Probably of limited value in adjustment disorders
Concentration on core concepts	Acceptance that a large number of disorders in DSM and ICD have limited validity and sustainability	Stress concept is a core one that is amenable to this model
Flexibility in accommodating new concepts	Need to change from overemphasis on specific DSM disorders so as to allow the evaluation of new ideas that may be of much greater heuristic value	The concept of adjustment disorders could certainly benefit from this approach, but only if there was a new understanding of how stress-related disorders are generated

So where are we now with ADs? What is abundantly clear is that ADs are very common, certainly more common than PTSD in most settings, and that nosologists likely would be much less preoccupied with operational criteria if researchers took the whole range of stress disorders into account before (usually wrongly) identifying certain features such as flashbacks and recurrent memories as being specific to only one group of disorders. The lack of specificity of the diagnosis of PTSD illustrated by Mol et al. (2005) supports the RDoC position that far too much attention is being given to the phenomenology and behavior associated with stress disorders and that the domain approach is the right way forward.

THE PLACE OF TRAUMA- AND STRESSOR-RELATED DISORDERS IN DSM-5 AND BEYOND

Two things are clear from this analysis of the present position of ADs in psychiatric classification. The first is that the phenomenology of stress and trauma is insufficient for diagnosis. It is a handmaiden for the clinician, not a signpost to understanding. The second is the need for an independent measure of stress, preferably a neurobiological one, that is uncontaminated by the nature of precipitating factors in the behavioral response. In the search for such a measure, the role of personality seems to be important. Individuals with personality dysfunction have a much lower threshold for pathological responses to stress than do those who have no personality problems. The consequence is that people with personality disorder have much more frequent episodes of apparent ADs because they are much more vulnerable to the effects of even minor stress (Seivewright et al. 2000). However, by changing the diagnostic criteria for ADs, those individuals with more prominent personality problems are excluded and the condition might appear to be less associated than it really is. The architects of DSM-III were aware of this issue when they formulated the diagnostic criteria for AD, and by excluding from the diagnosis those patients who have had recurrent symptomatology in response to minor stress, at a stroke they removed many patients from the diagnosis whose primary diagnosis was a personality disorder, although they probably should have been included.

Many years ago, Jeffrey Gray (1982) postulated that anxiety was generated when there was a mismatch between expected and actual stimuli presenting to the afferent pathways of the nervous system, particularly in the amygdala. Unfortunately, this theory has remained at the theoretical rather than experimental level, and the field is in urgent need of a breakthrough here. If indeed there is an independent index of stress in the nervous system, it would revolutionize the understanding of this group of disorders and lead to a completely different form of classification. To take an example from the field of botany, for 200 years plants have been classified by their morphological characteristics, especially their reproductive ones. With the discovery that DNA sequencing shows a completely different interrelationship between the families of plants, the whole system of classification is having to be altered. The morphological system of classification will be replaced by one that reduces plants to their essential elements. The same type of discovery is necessary for stress.

Key Points

- Phenomenology is generally not helpful in the diagnosis of adjustment disorders (ADs).

- Clinical judgment is a key element in making the diagnosis of ADs because it aims to balance the relative influences of resilience, stress, and symptomatology.

- Past personality status is highly relevant in the understanding of ADs.

- The Research Domain Criteria system of diagnosis has the potential to help in understanding the fundamental nature of stress disorders by taking them together as a general domain rather than as specific diagnoses.

- It is not especially helpful to consider ADs as subsyndromal conditions of lower importance.

- Operational criteria are of very limited value in understanding ADs.

- Stress needs to be understood much more at a neurophysiological level if diagnosis is to become more accurate.

- The differentiation of posttraumatic stress disorders (PTSD) from ADs should not be determined just by the presence or absence of traumatic experience.

- The required number and form of symptoms for the diagnosis of PTSD are probably too broad in DSM, and more harmony with ICD-11 would be helpful to reduce overdiagnosis.

- An independent measure of stress would be invaluable.

SUGGESTED READINGS

Rosen GM, Frueh C (eds): Clinician's Guide to Posttraumatic Stress Disorder. New York, Wiley, 2010

Tyrer P: Models for Mental Disorder, 5th Edition. New York, Wiley, 2013

REFERENCES

American Psychiatric Association: Diagnostic and Statistical Manual of Mental Disorders, 3rd Edition. Washington, DC, American Psychiatric Association, 1980

American Psychiatric Association: Diagnostic and Statistical Manual of Mental Disorders, 4th Edition. Washington, DC, American Psychiatric Association, 1994

American Psychiatric Association: Diagnostic and Statistical Manual of Mental Disorders, 5th Edition. Arlington, VA, American Psychiatric Association, 2013

Cooper JE, Kendell RE, Gurland BJ, et al: Psychiatric Diagnosis in New York and London. London, Oxford University Press, 1972

Craddock N, Mynors-Wallis L: Psychiatric diagnosis: impersonal, imperfect and important. Br J Psychiatry 204(2):93–95, 2014 24493652

Cuthbert BN, Insel TR: Toward the future of psychiatric diagnosis: the seven pillars of RDoC. BMC Med 11:126, 2013 23672542

Doherty AM, Jabbar F, Kelly BD, et al: Distinguishing between adjustment disorder and depressive episode in clinical practice: the role of personality disorder. J Affect Disord 168:78–85, 2014 25043318

Feighner JP, Robins E, Guze SB: Diagnostic criteria for use in psychiatric research. Arch Gen Psychiatry 26(1):57–63, 1972 5009428

Forbes D, Lockwood E, Creamer M, et al: Latent structure of the proposed ICD-11 post-traumatic stress disorder symptoms: implications for the diagnostic algorithm. Br J Psychiatry 206(3):245–251, 2015 25573397

Frances A: Saving Normal: An Insider's Revolt Against Out-of-Control Psychiatric Diagnosis, DSM-5, Big Pharma, and the Medicalization of Ordinary Life. New York, William Morrow, 2013

Gray JA: The Neuropsychology of Anxiety: An Enquiry Into the Function of the Septo-Hippocampal System. London, Oxford University Press, 1982

Guze SB: The role of follow-up studies: their contribution to diagnostic classification as applied to hysteria. Semin Psychiatry 2(4):392–402, 1970 5527407

Guze SB, Woodruff RA, Clayton PJ: A study of conversion symptoms in psychiatric outpatients. Am J Psychiatry 128:643–646, 1971

Guze SB, Cloninger CR, Martin RL, et al: A follow-up and family study of Briquet's syndrome. Br J Psychiatry 149:17–23, 1986 3779275

Insel TR: The NIMH Research Domain Criteria (RDoC) Project: precision medicine for psychiatry. Am J Psychiatry 171(4):395–397, 2014 24687194

Jaspers K: Allgemeine psychopathologie (1913), in General Psychopathology, Volumes 1 and 2. Translated by Hoenig J, Hamilton MW. Baltimore, MD, Johns Hopkins University Press, 1997, pp 381–394

Kupfer DJ: Introduction, in A Research Agenda for DSM-V. Edited by Kupfer J, First MB, Regier DA (eds). Washington, DC, American Psychiatric Press, 2002, pp xv–xxiii

McHugh PR, Slavney PR: Mental illness—comprehensive evaluation or checklist? N Engl J Med 366(20):1853–1855, 2012 22591291

Mol SS, Arntz A, Metsemakers JF, et al: Symptoms of post-traumatic stress disorder after non-traumatic events: evidence from an open population study. Br J Psychiatry 186:494–499, 2005 15928360

O'Donnell ML, Alkemade N, Nickerson A, et al: Impact of the diagnostic changes to post-traumatic stress disorder for DSM-5 and the proposed changes to ICD-11. Br J Psychiatry 205(3):230–235, 2014 24809400

Paris J: The Intelligent Clinician's Guide to the DSM-5. New York, Oxford University
    Press, 2013
Seivewright H, Tyrer P, Johnson T: Prediction of outcome in neurotic disorder: a 5-year
    prospective study. Psychol Med 28(5):1149–1157, 1998 9794022
Seivewright N, Tyrer P, Ferguson B, et al: Longitudinal study of the influence of life
    events and personality status on diagnostic change in three neurotic disorders. De-
    press Anxiety 11(3):105–113, 2000 10875051
Sharpe L, Gurland BJ, Fleiss JL, et al: Comparisons of American, Canadian and British
    psychiatrists in their diagnostic concepts. Can Psychiatr Assoc J 19(3):235–245,
    1974 4842273
Tyrer P, Seivewright H, Johnson T: The Nottingham Study of Neurotic Disorder: predic-
    tors of 12-year outcome of dysthymic, panic and generalized anxiety disorder. Psy-
    chol Med 34(8):1385–1394, 2004 15724870
Tyrer P, Reed GM, Crawford MJ: Classification, assessment, prevalence, and effect of
    personality disorder. Lancet 385(9969):717–726, 2015 25706217

Conceptual Framework and Controversies in Adjustment Disorders

JAMES J. STRAIN, M.D.
PATRICIA R. CASEY, M.D., F.R.C.PSYCH.

TRAUMA- AND stressor-related disorders, a new diagnostic class in DSM-5 (American Psychiatric Association 2013), includes the disorders in which exposure to a traumatic or stressful event is listed specifically as a diagnostic criterion. These include 1) reactive attachment disorder, 2) disinhibited social engagement disorder, 3) posttraumatic stress disorder (PTSD), 4) acute stress disorder (ASD), 5) adjustment disorders (ADs), and 6) other specified trauma- and stressor-related disorders. The first two disorders apply to children and are not discussed in this book. This chapter focuses on the seminal changes made from DSM-IV-TR in the last four of these disorders (American Psychiatric Association 2000) to DSM-5.

The organizers of DSM-5 decided that these disorders should be combined because of the commonality of their being precipitated by a stressor (*traumatic* or *nontraumatic*)—that is, etiology—rather than common symptoms—that is, phenomenology. As a result of literature reviews, examination of recent research studies, and consultant discussions, the decision was made to remove PTSD and ASD from the anxiety group and to move ADs to join the genre of other stressor-related diagnoses rather than remaining as a free-standing, residual, solitary-placement diagnosis (Strain and Friedman 2011). Many patients who have

PTSD and ASD do not have a fear-based syndrome, but instead "the most prominent clinical characteristics are anhedonic and dysphoric symptoms, externalizing angry and aggressive symptoms, or dissociative symptoms" (American Psychiatric Association 2013, p. 265). The organizers of DSM-5 felt that there were both heuristic value and clinical utility in grouping specific diagnoses within broad organizing diagnostic categories. By placing ADs with other primary psychiatric disorders, they encouraged the idea that its status as a residual or subthreshold diagnosis would be changed (Box 3–1).

Box 3–1.   DSM-5 Diagnostic Criteria for Adjustment Disorders

---

A. The development of emotional or behavioral symptoms in response to an identifiable stressor(s) occurring within 3 months of the onset of the stressor(s).
B. These symptoms or behaviors are clinically significant, as evidenced by one or both of the following:
   1. Marked distress that is out of proportion to the severity or intensity of the stressor, taking into account the external context and the cultural factors that might influence symptom severity and presentation.
   2. Significant impairment in social, occupational, or other important areas of functioning.
C. The stress-related disturbance does not meet the criteria for another mental disorder and is not merely an exacerbation of a preexisting mental disorder.
D. The symptoms do not represent normal bereavement.
E. Once the stressor or its consequences have terminated, the symptoms do not persist for more than an additional 6 months.

Specify whether:
   309.0 (F43.21) With depressed mood: Low mood, tearfulness, or feelings of hopelessness are predominant.
   309.24 (F43.22) With anxiety: Nervousness, worry, jitteriness, or separation anxiety is predominant.
   309.28 (F43.23) With mixed anxiety and depressed mood: A combination of depression and anxiety is predominant.
   309.3 (F43.24) With disturbance of conduct: Disturbance of conduct is predominant.
   309.4 (F43.25) With mixed disturbance of emotions and conduct: Both emotional symptoms (e.g., depression, anxiety) and a disturbance of conduct are predominant.
   309.9 (F43.20) Unspecified: For maladaptive reactions that are not classifiable as one of the specific subtypes of adjustment disorder.

Although dissociative disorders commonly occur following adverse occurrences, they do not require a specified stressor as a criterion and consequently are grouped in a separate diagnostic class in DSM-5. That is, stressors for the dissociative disorders are identified not as *etiological* or *precipitating* agents but rather as *predisposing* elements (Friedman et al. 2011). (Dissociative disorders are discussed more completely in Chapter 7, "Disintegrated Experience.")

DSM-5 PTSD criteria include four major symptom clusters—reexperiencing, avoidance, persistent negative alterations in cognitions and mood, and alterations in arousal and reactivity. The fourth cluster retains most DSM-IV-TR arousal symptoms but also includes "irritable behavior or angry outbursts and reckless or self-destructive behavior" (American Psychiatric Association 2013, p. 812). (PTSD is reviewed at length in Chapter 6, "Posttraumatic Stress Disorder.")

ASD was first employed in DSM-IV (American Psychiatric Association 1994) to demarcate acute stress reactions that occur in the initial month after exposure to a "traumatic" event and before the possibility of diagnosing PTSD (which requires a duration of 1 month after the stressor occurs) and to identify trauma survivors in the acute phase who were thought to be at high risk for PTSD. The evidence suggests that ASD does not adequately identify most patients who will develop PTSD (Bryant et al. 2011). Instead, ASD should be reserved for acute stress disorders that occur during the 3–30 day period after the occurrence of the traumatic stressor. The nature of the traumatic stressor is specified in Criterion A of DSM-5. Criterion B requires the presence of nine or more symptoms from five categories: intrusion, negative mood, dissociation, avoidance, and arousal. These criteria clearly differentiate ASD from the ADs, which are precipitated by a traumatic or nontraumatic stressor and do not require the Criterion B symptom profile. Also, ADs have both an acute form (less than 6 months) and a chronic form (6 months or longer) and are not restricted by the 3- to 30-day limitation of ASD. (ASD is discussed in depth in Chapter 5, "Acute Stress Disorder.")

ICD-10, in contrast to DSM-IV, describes an acute stress *reaction* (rather than *disorder*) as a transient reaction that can be evident *immediately* after the traumatic event and usually resolves within 2–3 days thereafter (World Health Organization 1992). Therefore, an acute stress reaction begins before ASD can be diagnosed (after symptoms have persisted for at least 3 days). It may be that those patients whose symptoms last beyond 3 days rather than ending by day 3 are a different cohort. Also, during the first 3 days, a DSM-5 diagnosis of an AD may be used before the diagnosis is revised to ASD if appropriate.

HISTORY AND EVOLUTION OF DSM ADJUSTMENT DISORDERS

Table 3–1 lists the diagnoses for what are now called ADs that were used in all DSM editions through DSM-IV-TR (American Psychiatric Association 1952, 1968, 1980, 1987, 1994, 2000). The diagnosis of AD has undergone a major evolution since DSM-I, in which it was referred to as a "transient situational personality disorder."

Furthermore, in DSM-IV-TR the term *psychosocial stressor* was changed to the broader concept of *stressor*. This change was made to take account of the fact that not all stressors leading to ADs were psychosocial. For example, surgery is associated with ADs (Oxman et al. 1994), and ADs were also found to be a common diagnosis in survivors of the Chernobyl reactor incident (Havenaar et al. 1996). A further step in the historical evolution of ADs has come about with their placement in the new trauma- and stressor-related disorders diagnostic class in DSM-5. This is a welcome occurrence because placing ADs in the same group as PTSD and ASD is likely to focus greater attention on and increase research into this condition and ultimately lead to its being viewed as a primary diagnosis.

In DSM-IV, the term *not otherwise specified* (NOS) was used for subthreshold disorders. Because of overuse of the NOS categories, this diagnosis was removed from the individual categories in DSM-5 and instead attached to each major grouping as "other specified disorder" and "unspecified disorder." DSM-5 describes other specified trauma- and stressor-related disorder as follows: "This category applies to presentations in which symptoms characteristic of a trauma- and stressor-related disorder that cause clinically significant distress or impairment in social, occupational, or other important areas of functioning predominate but do not meet the full criteria for any of the disorders in [this] diagnostic class" (American Psychiatric Association 2013, p. 289).

Historically, subthreshold PTSD and ASD were classified as ADs because they failed to reach the diagnostic threshold for the full disorder. During the development of DSM-5, consideration was given to continuing this diagnostic niche within ADs but to designate subthreshold PTSD and ASD as subtypes of ADs along with the preexisting subtypes. If implemented, this change would have meant that the traditional subtypes based on symptoms (depression, anxiety, conduct disturbance, or mixed) would have been augmented by subtypes based on traumatic stressors and discrete symptoms (ASD and PTSD subtypes). This would have facilitated comparative study of vulnerability and resilience factors in these trauma-based subtypes compared with the more general subtypes exposed to nontraumatic stressors such as interpersonal or financial events. Comparative studies of these subthreshold groups with the full-blown disorders (Friedman et al. 2011; Strain and Friedman 2014) would also have been possible. Ultimately,

TABLE 3–1.	DSM classifications of adjustment disorders, 1952–2000

DSM-I (1952): Transient situational personality disorder

Gross stress reaction

Adult situational reaction

Adjustment reaction of infancy

Adjustment reaction of childhood

Adjustment reaction of adolescence

Adjustment reaction of late life

Other transient situational personality disturbance

DSM-II (1968): Transient situational disturbance

Adjustment reaction of infancy

Adjustment reaction of childhood

Adjustment reaction of adolescence

Adjustment reaction of late life

DSM-III (1980): Adjustment disorder

Adjustment disorder with depressed mood

Adjustment disorder with anxious mood

Adjustment disorder with mixed emotional features

Adjustment disorder with disturbance of conduct

Adjustment disorder with mixed disturbance of emotions and conduct

Adjustment disorder with work (or academic) inhibition

Adjustment disorder with withdrawal

Adjustment disorder with atypical features

DSM-III-R (1987): Adjustment disorder

Adjustment disorder with depressed mood

Adjustment disorder with anxious mood

Adjustment disorder with mixed emotional features

Adjustment disorder with disturbance of conduct

Adjustment disorder with mixed disturbance of emotions and conduct

Adjustment disorder with work (or academic) inhibition

Adjustment disorder with withdrawal

Adjustment disorder with physical complaints

Adjustment disorder not otherwise specified

TABLE 3–1.   DSM classifications of adjustment disorders, 1952–2000 *(continued)*

DSM-IV (1994) and DSM-IV-TR (2000): Adjustment disorders

Adjustment disorder with depressed mood

Adjustment disorder with anxiety

Adjustment disorder with mixed anxiety and depressed mood

Adjustment disorder with disturbance of conduct

Adjustment disorder with mixed disturbance of emotions and conduct

Adjustment disorder unspecified

---

the overseers of DSM-5 did not agree to this change, and instead these subthreshold categories are now included among the *other specified trauma- and stressor-related disorders.* Within this new category, all presentations, which may represent any of the five primary subthreshold trauma- and stressor-related disorders, are coded with the same code (309.89); there is no provision for individual code numbers.

Examples of the subthreshold conditions included in this "other" group in DSM-5 (American Psychiatric Association 2013, p. 289) are

1. adjustment-like disorders with delayed onset of symptoms that occur more than 3 months after the stressor
2. adjustment-like disorders with prolonged duration of more than 6 months without prolonged duration of the stressor
3. culture-bound conditions such as *ataque de nervios*
4. individuals who do not fulfill all the criteria for PTSD and ASD because those primary diagnoses do not have a partial or subthreshold PTSD or ASD subtype option within DSM-5
5. persistent complex bereavement disorder (for further discussion of grief, see the subsection "The Bereavement Exclusion" in this chapter and Chapter 8, "Persistent Complex Bereavement Disorder and Its Treatment")

A similar new category, *unspecified trauma- and stressor-related disorder,* is used to code conditions if the clinician chooses not to specify the reasons why the criteria are not met or if there is insufficient information to make a more specific diagnosis.

APPLYING THE CRITERIA IN CLINICAL PRACTICE

Clinical judgment plays a significant role in diagnosing ADs. Many questions arise: What is the definition of a stressor? How does the clinician determine what is clinically significant? What is a normal response to the circumstances in question? For example, Powell and McCone (2004), in their case report of a patient with an AD secondary to the September 11, 2001 terrorist attacks, highlight the problem of establishing what constitutes a normal response to a terrorist attack. Also, the diagnosis must take into account a person's age, culture, and personality factors (e.g., degree of neuroticism). Finally, the complex interplay between external events and internal resources (e.g., resilience) varies considerably from one individual to the next, so one person's threat is another's challenge (Charney 2004). (Resilience is discussed further in Chapter 9, "Therapeutic Adaptations of Resilience.")

CONTROVERSIES REGARDING ADJUSTMENT DISORDERS

ADs and the other stress-related disorders considered in this book are very different conceptually from most of the other mental disorders classified in DSM-5 because they are based on etiology—that is, the close temporal relationship to a stressful or traumatic event. ADs specifically also have a longitudinal component in that spontaneous resolution or improvement with the passage of time is part of the definition. Most other disorders are classified according to symptom thresholds and not etiology or course, often because the causative mechanism is not yet known. However, a number of controversies exist in relation to ADs, as discussed in the following subsections.

Specificity Versus Nonspecificity

Critics of the current approach to the AD diagnosis state that the symptom complex is too subjective or dependent on clinical judgment in contrast to sound operational criteria (Baumeister and Kufner 2009; Baumeister et al. 2009; Casey et al. 2006). In DSM-III (American Psychiatric Association 1980), ADs were deliberately designed to be phenomenologically nonspecific (Strain and Friedman 2011). The only requirement is alteration in mood, anxiety, *or* conduct (or combinations of these) that is associated with distress and/or dysfunction in work, or school, or relationships in excess of what would be culturally acceptable for the stressor involved. Indeed, diagnoses of ADs are based on subjective assessments with no objective guidelines as to when the symptoms or behaviors can be counted as criteria. Furthermore, ADs can be characterized by type: depressive, anxious, conduct disturbance, or mixed moods and behaviors. This nonspecificity is in marked contrast to the proposal by Maercker et al. (2007, 2013) for ADs in ICD-11, which requires *both* distress and dysfunction and two specific symptoms: 1) failure to adapt and 2) preoccupation with the stressor and should occur within *1 month* of the occurrence of the stressor (see Chapter 11, "ICD-10, ICD-11, and DSM-5"). Thus, ADs have been reconceptualized in DSM-5 as a stress response syndrome so that they fit into a theoretical context that places ADs at one end of the spectrum and PTSD and ASD at the other.

This nonspecificity has had great clinical utility because it offers a diagnosis for those patients who have significant clinical distress or dysfunction, and therefore qualify for psychiatric care, but who do not meet the criteria for other DSM-5 diagnoses. The nonspecific diagnosis has a diagnostic code for billing, which increases the chance that a patient will seek care. This diagnosis also allows for the identification of prodromal expressions of more primary disorders that are in early stages and could benefit from clinical intervention (Strain and Friedman 2011). This can be likened to prediabetic or prehypertensive states seen in medical disorders in that they represent an intermediate phase between normal functioning and pathology, as adumbrated in Chapter 1, "Borderline Between Normal and Pathological Responses." Additionally, as more data become available, these early states are constantly being refined, and the boundaries between normal, prodromal, and pathological states are being recalibrated.

On the other hand, ADs are one of the few disorders in DSM that are so loosely described despite being one of the most common disorders. Apart from the requirement that a stressor must act as a symptom trigger that results in dysfunction or distress, there are no other specified defining features except the accompanying mood or conduct disturbance. If the recommendations for more specific diagnostic criteria are accepted by the ICD-11 working group, then the ICD-11 approach to ADs will differ significantly from that of DSM-5 even though ADs are grouped among the trauma- and stressor-related disorders in both classification systems (Maercker et al. 2013).

The issue relating to the absence of specific criteria is complex. Although the nonspecificity has conferred a high level of utility on the AD diagnosis, this very usefulness—with ADs ranking as the seventh most frequently used diagnosis in a global sample of psychiatrists studied by the World Health Organization (Reed et al. 2013)—may be one of the reasons that many psychiatrists now feel that the time has come to operationalize its criteria and ultimately to stimulate research into this underexplored diagnosis.

Boundary Disputes

ADs lie in the diagnostic space between normal stress responses and common disorders such as major depression, generalized anxiety disorder, and PTSD. Although major depression and generalized anxiety disorder are frequently triggered by life events, such events are not essential criteria for these diagnoses, whereas such events are an integral part of the diagnosis of ADs. Conceptually, the AD diagnosis is based on etiology and longitudinal course, whereas most other psychiatric diagnoses, with the exception of other trauma- and stressor-induced diagnoses and substance use disorders, are diagnosed on the basis of symptom thresholds and duration. The diagnosis of ADs can be clinically challenging (see Chapter 4, "Adjustment Disorders").

The first boundary dispute involves the problem of distinguishing between ADs and normal adaptive stress reactions (Casey et al. 2001). Indeed, when the decision was first made to add ADs to DSM-III, one of the objections was that doing so would medicalize problems of living (Fabrega et al. 1987). The argument was that the diagnosis does not allow the clinician to decide whether the person is or is not ill because it does not conform to the approach used for most other psychiatric disorders (e.g., inclusion of a specific symptom profile). As discussed in the previous subsection, "Specificity Versus Nonspecificity," including specific diagnostic criteria might assist in making this distinction.

An important aspect of the AD diagnostic criteria is that symptoms must cause significant distress or functional impairment. Although all other DSM-IV disorders required these criteria, these disorders also included additional specific symptom clusters which theoretically aid in differentiating disorder from nondisorder. This is why several investigators (Baumeister and Kufner 2009; Casey et al. 2001; Maercker et al. 2007) recommended raising the bar for Criterion B (the distress-impairment criterion) for ADs by stipulating that affected individuals should exhibit *both* significant distress *and* functional impairment to meet AD diagnostic criteria. This recommendation was prompted by a concern that without a more stringent Criterion B, there was a risk of overpathologizing normal reactions to distressing events. The argument against raising the bar higher for ADs was that there was no empirical justification for doing so; no studies have examined the prevalence of ADs with the current Criterion B versus the more stringent proposed criterion. Because the entire DSM-5 approach stipulated that there should be a very high threshold for any modification and that proposed changes should be based on sufficient and substantial empirical evidence, the decision was to not change Criterion B. Therefore, the requirement remains for *either* significant distress *or* functional impairment.

The second boundary dispute involves distinguishing between ADs and major depression or between ADs and generalized anxiety disorder because clinically there is symptom overlap in both cases, although the latter differentiation has received little attention. Studies examining the symptom overlap between ADs and major depression have had inconsistent results; some researchers have found no difference in severity or type between the two disorders (Casey et al. 2006), whereas others have identified greater severity of depressive symptoms in individuals with major depression (Fernández et al. 2012). These varied findings might suggest that ADs are correctly seen as a subthreshold disorder occupying a position between normal reactions to stress and major depression or generalized anxiety disorder. However, the depression scores of individuals with ADs in the study by Fernández and colleagues averaged in the moderate range of severity. Personality disorder differs also between those with ADs and major depression, with the disorder being more common in the latter (Doherty et al. 2014). Further studies examining symptom distinctions between the two categories with a much larger sample are currently under way (P. C. Casey, personal communication, 2015).

Even if there are no symptom differences except severity between the two groups, are there other distinctions between them? ADs are the most common diagnosis among patients presenting with deliberate self-harm, and there are some features in this self-harm that separate ADs from major depression (Casey et al. 2015). Suicidal behavior occurs earlier in the course of ADs compared with major depression (Polyakova et al. 1998), and suicidal ideation occurs at a lower symptom threshold in patients with ADs; however, measures of suicide intent do not distinguish the groups (Casey et al. 2015). The interval from suicidal communication to self-harm is shorter (Runeson et al. 1996) in individuals with ADs than in those with major depression.

The sociodemographic profile and childhood risk variables (Polyakova et al. 1998) also differ between the two groups. In addition, readmission rates for patients with ADs are significantly lower than for those with major depression, generalized anxiety, or dysthymia (Jones et al. 2002), and hospitalization is shorter (Greenberg et al. 1995). Further research, both clinical and biological, is needed to assist clinicians in distinguishing ADs from other common mental disorders.

Subthreshold Versus Threshold Psychopathology

The AD diagnosis has clinical appeal to both doctors and patients. Compared with an idiopathic pathological psychiatric state, temporary emotional symptoms resulting directly from a stressful life event are viewed as a more normal human reaction and therefore as less stigmatizing. Additionally, the disorder's more benign course (especially in adults) encourages clinicians to be more optimistic prognostically (Slavney 1999). This optimism is shared by medical insurance carriers, who do not consider the diagnosis to be a preexisting condition. Notwithstanding these benefits, the issue of ADs' subthreshold status raises some concerns. The first of these relates to the position held by some that ADs should be a full-threshold disorder, and the second relates to the danger of confusing other subthreshold disorders with ADs and thus deflating ADs' actual prevalence in epidemiological studies.

Should ADs Be a Full-Threshold Disorder?

At present ADs cannot be diagnosed if the symptoms are best explained by another diagnosis. However, it is important to remember that the AD diagnosis can be used with another diagnosis that is comorbid. The complexity of diagnosis is illustrated by the following case vignette.

Case Vignette

Ms. A, a 60-year-old woman with no prior psychiatric history, has unexpectedly lost her job and is so upset at the financial hardship this causes that she has trouble sleeping, is constantly tired, cries frequently, has an increased appetite, and feels useless. She sees little hope of getting a job in the future because of her age. One month after the event, her concerned family members persuade her to visit her family doctor.

If Ms. A had gone to her doctor on day 10, following the onset of symptoms, she would have met the criteria for an AD because she had clinically significant symptoms (dysfunction) by virtue of their persistence and severity (noticed by family) that were triggered by the stressor of losing her job. The very close temporal relationship between the stressor and the onset of symptoms (dysfunction) suggests that if she found a new job, her symptoms would improve. However, by visiting her doctor after day 14, she would be diagnosed with major depression and probably given a prescription for antidepressants. Ms. A cannot be diagnosed with an AD because she has reached the symptom and duration threshold for major depression even though clinically the etiology and course of her symptoms suggest that AD is a more appropriate diagnosis even after 2 weeks.

DSM-5 recognizes the importance of clinical judgment, but it is unclear in a case like Ms. A's whether clinical judgment or the strict application of the DSM criteria should take precedence. If the context and timeline of symptoms were given more weight in DSM, this issue would be less problematic and ADs could still be diagnosed clinically even on day 14 and beyond. In a case such as Ms. A's, and as the criteria are currently framed, there is a danger that the "checkbox approach" based on symptom numbers will apply (McHugh and Slavney 2012) rather than the broader focus that is grounded in clinical judgment.

Because ADs are a subthreshold disorder, they are viewed as "mild" by many clinicians, as reflected in the following statement: "ADs are generally milder, more vaguely defined maladaptive responses to stressors that are broader in range than the A criterion of ASD and PTSD, from relatively mild to severe" (Friedman et al. 2011, p. 744). Technically, this is the correct conceptualization of a disorder that has not reached the threshold for a full-blown disorder. Longitudinal studies suggest a good prognosis in adults; however, in some countries ADs are the most common diagnosis associated with suicide (Manoranjitham et al. 2010) and are the most common diagnosis made in those engaging in self-harm behavior (Taggart et al. 2006). The finding that there are differences between major depression and ADs with respect to suicidal behavior and sociodemographic and childhood risk factors (see the earlier subsection "Boundary Disputes" and Chapter 1, "Borderline Between Normal and Pathological Responses"), as well as the fact that ADs culminate in suicide in some patients, suggests that consideration should be given to removing the subthreshold status of ADs and regarding them as a full-threshold disorder. It is likely that ICD-11 will be silent on this, thereby implicitly suggesting that ADs have full-threshold status (see Chapter 11).

Potential for Confusing Other Subthreshold Conditions and ADs

Subthreshold disorders occupy the borderland between normal and pathological reactions to stress. DSM-5, like its predecessors, regards individuals who do not reach the threshold for a specific disorder as having a subthreshold condition, and these individuals continue to fall within the provenance of a mental health condition. In the scientific literature various epithets have been applied to these conditions, including minor depression, subclinical depression, subsyndromal depression, subsyndromal symptomatic depression, and nonspecific depressive symptoms.

The heterogeneity of terms and definitions for minor and subthreshold conditions was confirmed in a systematic review by Rodríguez et al. (2012). *Subthreshold depression* was defined in most cases as depressed mood or loss of interest but with fewer than five symptoms or no significant impairment. With respect to *minor depression,* the highest level of agreement across studies was for no more than four symptoms lasting for a minimum of 2 weeks. *Subsyndromal symptomatic depression* was defined in most studies using the definition proposed by Judd et al. (1994): "any two or more simultaneous symptoms of depression, present for most or all of the time, at least two weeks in duration, associated with evidence of social dysfunction, occurring in individuals who do not meet criteria for diagnoses of minor depression, major depression, and/or dysthymia" (p. 18). Some definitions specifically excluded depressed mood or anhedonia, whereas others did not, and the minimum number of symptoms varied from two to five. From this study it is clear that the nosology used is diverse and highly confusing.

Surprisingly, mild depression is not a subthreshold condition but refers to major depression in which few if any symptoms are in excess of those required to meet the threshold for diagnosis. Moderate and severe forms of depression represent increases in the distress or dysfunction criteria.

What is the relevance of this heterogeneous terminology to the discussion of ADs? The point is that an individual could simultaneously meet the diagnostic criteria for ADs and for one or more of the subthreshold conditions described above. Such a situation is described in the following example.

Case Vignette

Mrs. P, a 40-year-old woman, experienced the breakup of her 10-year marriage 4 weeks ago. Since then she cries many times every day, has trouble going to work because of her distress, and has taken 3 days of sick leave. Because she lies awake for 2 hours at night, she has been given a prescription for hypnotics.

Mrs. P could be diagnosed with subsyndromal symptomatic depression ("any two or more simultaneous symptoms of depression, present for most or all of the time, at least two weeks in duration, associated with evidence of social dysfunction" [Judd et al. 1994, p. 18]) or with minor depression (requiring not more than four symptoms for 2 weeks) or with an AD (a subthreshold disorder in response to a stressful event), depending on whether the focus was on symptoms or etiology.

The potential for diagnostic confusion and ultimately the implications for the management of Mrs. P are obvious. This is particularly relevant because the main reason for identifying subthreshold disorders is the presumed need for treatment. However, the situation outlined in this vignette suggests that a person with an AD might require a more watchful approach to intervention. (Subthreshold diagnoses are also discussed in Chapter 1, "Borderline Between Normal and Pathological Responses.")

Subtypes of ADs

A question of relevance is whether all the AD subtypes listed in DSM-5 are necessary. DSM-5 includes ADs with depressed mood, with anxiety, with disturbance of conduct, and with mixed moods and behaviors. These subtypes have not been the subject of extensive research. Zimmerman et al. (2013) recommended that the anxious and depressed subtypes could be collapsed into one because no clinical or sociodemographic differences were identified between them; however, this study was limited in its methodology. This is an area needing much more research. (Note that the recommendation for ICD-11 is to eliminate subtypes. See Chapter 11.)

Additionally, other subtypes have been proposed. Suggestions that abnormal grief should be included as a subtype of ADs were rejected, and abnormal grief has been placed elsewhere in DSM-5 under the category persistent complex bereavement disorder. Calls for the inclusion of a new PTSD/ASD subtype of ADs, to accommodate individuals who do not meet the full criteria for either of these conditions, were also rejected by the DSM-5 Task Force, and such cases are diagnosed using the other specified trauma- and stressor-related disorder category.

The Bereavement Exclusion

The former DSM bereavement exclusion for major depression meant that if a person was recently bereaved, he or she could not be diagnosed with major depression. Now that this exclusion has been removed in DSM-5, it is possible in certain circumstances for a recently bereaved person to be diagnosed as having major depression (Kendler et al. 2008; Zisook et al. 2007). However, DSM-5 still retains the bereavement exclusion for ADs; Criterion D requires that the symptoms found "do not represent normal bereavement." DSM-5 states that the diagnosis of an AD may be made in certain bereavement situations "when the intensity, quality, or persistence of grief reactions exceeds what normally might be expected, when cultural, religious, or age-appropriate norms are taken into account" (American Psychiatric Association 2013, p. 287). It also states that "a more specific set of bereavement-related symptoms has been designated *persistent complex bereavement disorder*" (p. 287), which is classified among the other specified trauma- and stressor-related disorders (see Chapter 8).

The other specified trauma- and stressor-related disorder category creates a problem for clinicians and especially for bereavement researchers because this category is not subtyped, and the single category code (309.89) does not specify whether a presentation applies to PTSD, ASD, *ataque de nervios,* or persistent complex bereavement disorder. Therefore, it will not be possible to evaluate whether, for example, these abnormal grief reactions have the same course or symptom pattern as, say, subthreshold PTSD. The following case is an example of when this diagnosis might be used.

Case Vignette

Mrs. D lost her husband 18 months ago and has not been able to return to work or her exercise routine or meeting with friends. Most of the day she thinks of her departed husband and yearns for his return. She keeps his picture by her bed and constantly looks through the album of their combined photographs. She occasionally has a dream in which he has returned, but then she wakes up to find her bed empty. Mrs. D has neither removed his clothes from their shared closet nor sold his car, although she does not drive.

As described in DSM-5 the classification of persistent complex bereavement disorder both in ADs and in the other specified trauma- and stressor-related disorder category, without subtyping codes, is unsatisfactory and will have an adverse impact on research not just in relation to abnormal bereavement but also in relation to subthreshold PTSD and ASD. Ultimately, this situation will impede clarification of the clinical relevance of these syndromes because they cannot be differentiated from one another by codes.

Lack of Diagnostic Schedules and the Gold Standard

The difficulties related to the lack of specificity in the AD diagnosis signal the concerns about reliability and validity of the diagnosis; this lack of specificity may account for both the difficulty in crafting a measure for assessment of ADs and the lack of research for this diagnostic entity (Baumeister and Kufner 2009; Casey et al. 2006; Helmchen and Linden 2000). Most of the structured diagnostic interviews in common use do not assess ADs. The Schedules for Clinical Assessment in Neuropsychiatry (SCAN; World Health Organization 1994) and the Structured Clinical Interview for DSM-IV (SCID; First et al. 1996) include ADs but unsatisfactorily. In SCAN, ADs are located in Section 13, "Inferences and Attributions," which comes after the criteria for all other disorders have been completed and includes no specific questions to assist the interviewer in making the diagnosis. In SCID, the instructions to interviewers specify that this diagnosis is not made if the criteria for any other psychiatric disorder are met. An updated SCID for DSM-5—Clinician Version (SCID-5-CV) is available and will be helpful for deriving a more objective specification of the AD diagnosis (First et al. 2016; see Suggested Readings). The Mini International Neuropsychiatric Interview (MINI; Sheehan et al. 1998) also incorporates a section on ADs, but as in SCID, ADs are superseded when any other diagnosis is made. To our knowledge only two questionnaires have been developed for screening ADs, one by Einsle et al. (2010) and the other by Cornelius et al. (2014).

Such diagnostic tools are essential if there is to be effective research and the development of an evidence base that might inform future revisions of the AD criteria. The specific self-report measure developed by Einsle et al. (2010) for the purpose of identifying ADs is based on the theory of Maercker et al. (2007) that ADs, like PTSD, will feature certain symptoms that include three major symptom clusters. The self-rated questionnaire consists of 29 statements covering intrusions, avoidance, failure to adapt, anxiety, depression, and poor impulse control. In addition, a list of 29 stressors is presented for the individual to check as present or absent in the previous year and to identify the most prominent. This questionnaire has been used in several studies by Maercker et al. (2012), but at this point it has not been used more widely. One of the reasons for this lack of more widespread use is likely the measure's limited generalizability because it is based on a specific symptom model of ADs that closely resembles that of PTSD, and its use would eliminate many of the patients diagnosed with ADs using the DSM-5 criteria. Furthermore, it has not been replicated in diverse settings with diverse cohorts and populations.

A recent diagnostic instrument (Cornelius et al. (2014), the Diagnostic Interview Adjustment Disorder (DIAD), consists of 29 questions that identify the stressful event, the temporal relationship between stressor and symptoms, and the level of distress and impairment. The emergence of a new schedule to diagnose ADs is welcome, but it remains to be seen how well it performs in clinical studies and diverse populations.

The trained clinician remains the "gold standard" for diagnosis with the current DSM-5 AD taxonomy, enabling the differentiation of ADs from other psychiatric disorders.

PSYCHOBIOLOGICAL QUESTIONS IN ADJUSTMENT DISORDERS AND THE OTHER TRAUMA- AND STRESSOR-RELATED DISORDERS

Strain and Friedman (2011) reviewed the psychobiology that might apply to the ADs. A useful biological context within which the pathophysiology of depression, PTSD, anxiety disorders, and ADs is currently understood is that proposed by Hans Selye (1956) on the basis of his classic work on the key role of the hypothalamic-pituitary-adrenocortical (HPA) system in the human stress response. Such work has been updated by more sophisticated understanding of the neurocircuitry and psychobiological systems that mediate and moderate this response. Stress-induced alterations in HPA function are known to occur in depression, PTSD, and other anxiety disorders (Arborelius et al. 1999; Chrousos and Gold 1992; Kim and Gorman 2005; Southwick et al. 2007; Strohle and Holsboer 2003). Expanding on the suggestion by Maercker et al. (2007) to consider ADs as a stress response syndrome, it would be important to know how the HPA system operates in ADs and whether each AD subtype exhibits similar psychobiological alterations or is more similar to the parent mood state (e.g., depression, anxiety). With the extensive research (Dienstbier 1989) displaying stress-related HPA reactions, it is likely that at least some AD subtypes are associated with altered HPA mechanisms.

Chrousos and Gold (1992) and McEwen (2004) have examined the psychobiological differences between depression and chronic stress syndromes. Friedman and McEwen 2004) have done the same with respect to PTSD, as have others with regard to anxiety disorders (Arborelius et al. 1999; Strohle and Holsboer 2003). Overarching constructs such as allostatic load are useful in all cases (*allostatic load* has been conceptualized to refer to the wear and tear on the body that develops over time when an individual is exposed to chronic or repeated stress). Furthermore, there is considerable overlap between depression, PTSD, and certain anxiety disorders with regard to some associated biological (e.g., endocrine, cardiovascular, metabolic, and immunological) abnormalities. These relationships are far from perfect, however, and there may also be some differences between specific psychiatric disorders and chronic stress with regard to these findings. Extending this argument to ADs, it is unknown whether psychobiological abnormalities associated with depression will be seen in the AD depressive subtype and whether alterations found in anxiety disorders will be found in the AD anxiety subtype. Two fruitful lines of research are possible with regard to HPA function: 1) comparing AD subtypes with each other and 2) comparing specific AD subtypes (e.g., depressive subtype) with the parent disorder (e.g., depression).

Genetic findings regarding individual differences related to vulnerability and resilience may be another avenue to consider. Kilpatrick et al. (2007) demonstrated that individuals with the short allele of the serotonin transporter gene 5-HTTLPR who had high hurricane exposure and low social support were at greater risk for developing PTSD than a matched cohort with the long allele of this gene. This study replicates several trials regarding gene × environment interactions for depression (Caspi et al. 2003; Kaufman et al. 2004; Kilpatrick et al. 2007) and raises the critical question of vulnerability versus resilience for individuals exposed to stress, trauma, or depression. It has been shown that most people exposed to traumatic events or losses do not develop PTSD, depression, or anxiety disorders (Kessler et al. 1995). Although data are lacking, it is reasonable to suggest, by extension, that most people exposed to nontraumatic stressful events do not develop ADs or another psychiatric disorder. This raises a number of questions: Do the same genetic differences determine vulnerability versus resilience in depression, PTSD, other anxiety disorders, and ADs? Are the same psychobiological mechanisms involved (Charney 2004; Haglund et al. 2007)? Do people with ADs exhibit shared neural substrates, familiarity, genetic risk factors, environmental risk factors, biomarkers, temperamental antecedents, and/or abnormalities of cognitive or emotional processing with people with depression, PTSD, ASD, or other anxiety disorders? Finally, will treatments that effectively produce clinical remission in depression, anxiety disorders, PTSD, or ASD also be effective for the respective subtypes of ADs? Hopefully, the HPA heuristic may provide a useful psychobiological context within which to encourage both basic research and clinical trials that will enhance general understanding of the relationship between stress response syndromes, depression, anxiety disorders, PTSD, and ADs. In addition, such investigations should also provide a theoretical context within which to investigate different therapeutic approaches for the different AD subtypes.

CONCLUSION

Although ADs and their antecedents, such as transient situational personality disorder and transient situational disturbance, have been included as a diagnosis in DSM for more than half a century, they remain underresearched. Their overlap with other disorders, their subthreshold status, and their subtypes are all open to challenge and controversy. Nevertheless, ADs remain an important and useful diagnosis and, arguably, one that is less stigmatizing than others. There are more questions than answers with regard to ADs, and recent changes in the way they are classified may pave the way for much-needed research.

Key Points

- The diagnosis of an adjustment disorder (AD) requires the presence of a significant but not necessarily traumatic stressor, dysfunction, and dysphoria in excess of what would normally be expected in the patient's culture.

- Symptoms secondary to a medical illness may not be counted in the algorithm for the diagnosis of an AD.

- A new DSM-5 diagnostic category, other specified trauma- and stressor-related disorder, has been added to accommodate presentations involving different time dimensions, *ataque de nervios* and other cultural syndromes, and persistent complex bereavement disorder.

- Controversies surround when dysfunction, dysphoria, or a stressor is sufficient to support the diagnosis of an AD.

- The ADs are confounded by the degree of specificity versus nonspecificity accepted in the diagnosis.

- Normal grief is an exclusionary criterion for the ADs.

- The trained clinician remains the "gold standard" for diagnosis using the current DSM-5 criteria for ADs.

SUGGESTED READINGS

Casey P, Bailey S: Adjustment disorders: the state of the art. World Psychiatry 10(1):11–18, 2011 21379346

First MJ, Williams JBW, Karg RS, Spitzer RL: Structured Clinical Interview for DSM-5—Clinician Version (SCID-5-CV), Arlington, VA, American Psychiatric Association, 2016

Friedman MJ, Resick PA, Bryant RA, et al: Classification of trauma and stressor-related disorders in DSM-5. Depress Anxiety 28(9):737–749, 2011 21681870

Strain JJ, Friedman MJ: Considering adjustment disorders as stress response syndromes for DSM-5. Depress Anxiety 28(9):818–823, 2011 21254314

REFERENCES

American Psychiatric Association: Diagnostic and Statistical Manual: Mental Disorders. Washington, DC, American Psychiatric Association, 1952

American Psychiatric Association: Diagnostic and Statistical Manual of Mental Disorders, 2nd Edition. Washington, DC, American Psychiatric Association, 1968

American Psychiatric Association: Diagnostic and Statistical Manual of Mental Disorders, 3rd Edition. Washington, DC, American Psychiatric Association, 1980

American Psychiatric Association: Diagnostic and Statistical Manual of Mental Disorders, 3rd Edition, Revised. Washington, DC, American Psychiatric Association, 1987

American Psychiatric Association: Diagnostic and Statistical Manual of Mental Disorders, 4th Edition. Washington, DC, American Psychiatric Association, 1994

American Psychiatric Association: Diagnostic and Statistical Manual of Mental Disorders, 4th Edition, Text Revision. Washington, DC, American Psychiatric Association, 2000

American Psychiatric Association: Diagnostic and Statistical Manual of Mental Disorders, 5th Edition, Arlington, VA, American Psychiatric Association 2013

Arborelius L, Owens MJ, Plotsky PM, et al: The role of corticotropin-releasing factor in depression and anxiety disorders. J Endocrinol 160(1):1–12, 1999 9854171

Baumeister H, Kufner K: It is time to adjust the adjustment disorder category. Curr Opin Psychiatry 22(4):409–412, 2009 19436201

Baumeister H, Maercker A, Casey P: Adjustment disorder with depressed mood: a critique of its DSM-IV and ICD-10 conceptualisations and recommendations for the future. Psychopathology 42(3):139–147, 2009 19276640

Bryant RA, Friedman MJ, Spiegel D, et al: A review of acute stress disorder in DSM-5. Depress Anxiety 28(9):802–817, 2011 21910186

Casey P, Dowrick C, Wilkinson G: Adjustment disorders: fault line in the psychiatric glossary. Br J Psychiatry 179:479–481, 2001 11731347

Casey P, Maracy M, Kelly BD, et al: Can adjustment disorder and depressive episode be distinguished? Results from the ODIN study. J Affect Disord 92(2–3):291–297, 2006 16515807

Casey P, Jabbar F, O'Leary E, et al: Suicidal behaviors in adjustment disorder and depressive episode. J Affect Disord 174:441–446, 2015 25553405

Caspi A, Sugden K, Moffitt TE et al: Influence of life stress on depression: moderation by a polymorphism in the 5-IITT gene. Science 301(5631):386–389, 2003 12869766

Charney DS: Psychobiological mechanisms of resilience and vulnerability: implications for successful adaptation to extreme stress. Am J Psychiatry 161(2):195–216, 2004 14754765

Chrousos GP, Gold PW: The concepts of stress and stress system disorders: overview of physical and behavioral homeostasis. JAMA 267(9):1244–1252, 1992 1538563

Cornelius LR, Brouwer S, de Boer MR, et al: Development and validation of the Diagnostic Interview Adjustment Disorder (DIAD). Int J Methods Psychiatr Res 23(2):192–207, 2014 24478059

Dienstbier RA: Arousal and physiological toughness: implications for mental and physical health. Psychol Rev 96(1):84–100, 1989 2538855

Doherty AM, Jabbar F, Kelly BD, et al: Distinguishing between adjustment disorder and depressive episode in clinical practice: the role of personality disorder. J Affect Disord 168:78–85, 2014 25043318

Einsle F, Köllner V, Dannemann S, et al: Development and validation of a self-report for the assessment of adjustment disorders. Psychol Health Med 15(5):584–595, 2010 20835968

Fabrega HJr, Mezzich JE, Mezzich AC: Adjustment disorder as a marginal or transitional illness category in DSM-III. Arch Gen Psychiatry 44(6):567–572, 1987 3579503

Fernández A, Mendive JM, Salvador-Carulla L, et al; DASMAP investigators: Adjustment disorders in primary care: prevalence, recognition and use of services. Br J Psychiatry 201:137–142, 2012 22576725

First MJ, Spitzer RL, Gibbon M, Williams JBW: Structured Clinical Interview for DSM-IV Axis I Disorders, Clinician Version (SCID-CV). Washington, DC, American Psychiatric Press, 1996

First MJ, Williams JBW, Karg RS, Spitzer RL: Structured Clinical Interview for DSM-5—Clinician Version (SCID-5-CV). Arlington, VA, American Psychiatric Association, 2016

Friedman MJ, McEwen BS: Posttraumatic stress disorder, allostatic load, and medical illness, in Trauma and Health: Physical Consequences of Exposure to Extreme Stress. Edited by Schnurr PP, Green BI. Washington, DC, American Psychological Association, 2004, pp 157–188

Friedman MJ, Resick PA, Bryant RA, et al: Classification of trauma and stressor-related disorders in DSM-5. Depress Anxiety 28(9):737–749, 2011 21681870

Greenberg WM, Rosenfeld D, Ortega E: Adjustment disorder as an admission diagnosis. Am J Psychiatry 152(3):459–461, 1995 7864279

Haglund ME, Nestadt PS, Cooper NS, et al: Psychobiological mechanisms of resilience: relevance to prevention and treatment of stress-related psychopathology. Dev Psychopathol 19(3):889–920, 2007 17705907

Havenaar JM, Van den Brink W, Van den Bout J, et al: Mental health problems in the Gomel region (Belarus): an analysis of risk factors in an area affected by the Chernobyl disaster. Psychol Med 26(4):845–855, 1996 8817720

Helmchen H, Linden M: Subthreshold disorders in psychiatry: clinical reality, methodological artifact, and the double-threshold problem. Compr Psychiatry 41(2 suppl 1):1–7, 2000 10746897

Jones R, Yates WR, Zhou MH: Readmission rates for adjustment disorders: comparison with other mood disorders. J Affect Disord 71(1–3):199–203, 2002 12167517

Judd LL, Rapaport MH, Paulus MP et al: Subsyndromal symptomatic depression: a new mood disorder. J Clin Psychiatry 55(suppl):18–28, 1994 8077164

Kaufman J, Yang B-Z, Douglas-Palumberi H, et al: Social supports and serotonin transporter gene moderate depression in maltreated children. Proc Natl Acad Sci USA 101(49):17316–17321, 2004 15563601

Kendler KS, Myers J, Zisook S: Does bereavement-related major depression differ from major depression associated with other stressful life events? Am J Psychiatry 165(11):1449–1455, 2008 18708488

Kessler RC, Sonnega A, Bromet E, et al: Posttraumatic stress disorder in the National Comorbidity Survey. Arch Gen Psychiatry 52(12):1048–1060, 1995 7492257

Kilpatrick DG, Koenen KC, Ruggiero KJ, et al: The serotonin transporter genotype and social support and moderation of posttraumatic stress disorder and depression in hurricane-exposed adults. Am J Psychiatry 164(11):1693–1699, 2007 17974934

Kim J, Gorman J: The psychobiology of anxiety. Clin Neurosci Res 4:335–347, 2005

Maercker A, Einsle F, Kollner V: Adjustment disorders as stress response syndromes: a new diagnostic concept and its exploration in a medical sample. Psychopathology 40(3):135–146, 2007 17284941

Maercker A, Forstmeier S, Pielmaier L, et al: Adjustment disorders: prevalence in a representative nationwide survey in Germany. Soc Psychiatry Psychiatr Epidemiol 47(11):1745–1752, 2012 22407021

Maercker A, Brewin CR, Bryant RA, et al: Proposals for mental disorders specifically associated with stress in the International Classification of Diseases-11. Lancet 381(9878):1683–1685, 2013 23583019

Manoranjitham SD, Rajkumar AP, Thangadurai P, et al: Risk factors for suicide in rural south India. Br J Psychiatry 196(1):26–30, 2010 20044655

McEwen BS: Protection and damage from acute and chronic stress: allostasis and allostatic overload and relevance to the pathophysiology of psychiatric disorders. Ann NY Acad Sci 1032:1–7, 2004 15677391

McHugh PR, Slavney PR: Mental illness—comprehensive evaluation or checklist? N Engl J Med 366(20):1853–1855, 2012 22591291

Oxman TE, Barrett JE, Freeman DH, et al: Frequency and correlates of adjustment disorder related to cardiac surgery in older patients. Psychosomatics 35(6):557–568, 1994 7809358

Polyakova I, Knobler HY, Ambrumova A, et al: Characteristics of suicide attempts in major depression versus adjustment disorder. J Affect Disord 47(1–3):159–167, 1998 9476756

Powell S, McCone D: Treatment of AD with anxiety: a September 11, 2001, case study with a 1-year follow-up. Cogn Behav Pract 11:331–336, 2004

Reed GM, Roberts MC, Keeley J, et al: Mental health professionals' natural taxonomies of mental disorders: implications for the clinical utility of the ICD-11 and the DSM-5. J Clin Psychol 69(12):1191–1212, 2013 24122386

Rodríguez MR, Nuevo R, Chatterji S, et al: Definitions and factors associated with subthreshold depressive conditions: a systematic review. BMC Psychiatry 12:181, 2012 23110575

Runeson BS, Beskow J, Waern M: The suicidal process in suicides among young people. Acta Psychiatr Scand 93(1):35–42, 1996 8919327

Selye H: The Stress of Life. New York, McGraw-Hill, 1956

Sheehan D, Lecrubier Y, Sheehan KH, et al: The Mini-International Neuropsychiatric Interview (M.I.N.I.): the development and validation of a structured diagnostic psychiatric interview for DSM-IV and ICD-10. J Clin Psychiatry 59(suppl 20):22–33, quiz 34–57, 1998 9881538

Slavney PR: Diagnosing demoralization in consultation psychiatry. Psychosomatics 40(4):325–329, 1999 10402879

Southwick SM, Davis LL, Atkins ED, et al: Neurobiological alterations associated with PTSD, in Handbook of PTSD: Science and Practice. Edited by Friedman MJ, Keane TM, Resnick PA. New York, Guilford, 2007, pp 166–189

Strain JJ, Friedman MJ: Considering adjustment disorders as stress response syndromes for DSM-5. Depress Anxiety 28(9):818–823, 2011 21254314

Strain JJ, Friedman MJ: Adjustment disorders, in Gabbard's Treatment of Psychiatric Disorders, Fifth Edition. Edited by Gabbard GO. Washington, DC, American Psychiatric Publishing, 2014, pp 519–529

Strohle A, Holsboer F: Stress responsive neurohormones in depression and anxiety. Pharmacopsychiatry 36(suppl 3):207–214, 2003 14677081

Taggart C, O'Grady J, Stevenson M, et al: Accuracy of diagnosis at routine psychiatric assessment in patients presenting to an accident and emergency department. Gen Hosp Psychiatry 28(4):330–335, 2006 16814633

World Health Organization: International Statistical Classification of Diseases and Related Health Problems, 10th Revision. Geneva, World Health Organization, 1992

World Health Organization: Schedules for Clinical Assessment in Neuropsychiatry, Version 2.0 Manual. Geneva, World Health Organization, 1994

Zimmerman M, Martinez JH, Dalrymple K, et al: Is the distinction between adjustment disorder with depressed mood and adjustment disorder with mixed anxious and depressed mood valid? Ann Clin Psychiatry 25(4):257–265, 2013 24199215

Zisook S, Shear K, Kendler KS: Validity of the bereavement exclusion criterion for the diagnosis of major depressive episode. World Psychiatry 6(2):102–107, 2007

CHAPTER 4

Adjustment Disorders

EPIDEMIOLOGY, DIAGNOSIS, AND TREATMENT

James J. Strain, M.D.

THE PURPOSE of this chapter is to review the etiology, epidemiology, diagnosis, and especially treatment of the adjustment disorders (ADs). The background of these disorders sets the stage for a description of their treatment and management by clinicians.

ETIOLOGY

Stress is the etiological agent for ADs; however, diverse variables, modifiers, and features of resilience are involved that affect who will experience an AD following stress. It is important to underscore that a traumatic stressor is not required to precipitate an AD. Cohen (1981) argued that 1) acute stresses are different from chronic ones in both psychological and physiological terms; 2) the meaning of the stress is affected by "modifiers" (e.g., ego strengths, support systems, prior mastery, resilience, genetic predisposition); and 3) the manifest and latent meanings of the stressor(s) must be differentiated (e.g., a job loss may be a relief or a catastrophe). ADs with maladaptive denial of pregnancy, for example, can be a consequence of a stressor such as separation from a partner (Brezinka et al. 1994). An objectively overwhelming stressor may have little effect on one individual, whereas a minor one could be regarded as cataclysmic by another. A recent minor stress superimposed on a previous underlying (major) stress that had no observable effect on its own may have a significant additive effect and foster the outbreak of symptoms (i.e., concatenation of events) (B. Hamburg, personal communication, April 1990). The subjective meaning of the stressor is key to its effect on the alloplastic load on the individual. The meaning of the stressor and the concatenation of events that may proceed from a stressor are illustrated in the following example.

Case Vignette

Mr. T lost his job and then 3 months later defaulted on his mortgage and lost his house. His children have had to move to a lesser school district, and the family is now living in downscale public housing. Mr. T has both anxious and depressed feelings and intense worries about his and his family's future. He has no difficulty sleeping, however, and his appetite and energy have been close to normal.

Andreasen and Wasek (1980) observed the differences between the chronicity of stressors found in adolescents and those observed in adults: 59% and 35%, respectively, of the stressors had been present for 1 year or more and 9% and 39% for 3 months or less. Popkin et al. (1990) found that in 68.6% of the cases in their consultation-liaison cohort, a medical illness itself was judged to be the primary stressor. Snyder and Strain (1989) observed that stressors as assessed on Axis IV of DSM-IV (American Psychiatric Association 1994) were significantly higher ($P=0.0001$) for consultation-liaison patients with ADs than for patients with other diagnostic disorders, supporting the construct that a stressor was the mechanism triggering or at least associated with the AD.

Although more attention has been directed toward the current precipitating stressor in the diagnosis of ADs, some investigations have highlighted the role of childhood experiences in the vulnerability to these disorders. Several studies of young male soldiers with ADs secondary to conscription revealed that stressors at a young age, such as abusive or overprotective parenting or adverse early family events, are risk factors for the later development of ADs (For-Wey et al. 2002; Giotakos and Konstantakopoulos 2002). In a similar cohort, a history of childhood separation anxiety was also found to be associated with the later development of ADs (Kovacs et al. 1994).

PREVALENCE

ADs occur in children, adolescents, and elderly individuals (2%–8% in community samples) in acute care general hospital inpatients (12%), in mental health outpatient settings (10%–30%), and in special settings, such as following cardiac surgery (up to 50%) (Oxman et al. 1994). Adult women are given the diagnosis of ADs twice as often as adult men, but no gender difference has been found in adolescents and children (Fabrega et al. 1987). In a primary care study the prevalence of ADs was 2.9% when patients were assessed using the Structured Clinical Interview for DSM-IV (Fernández et al. 2012), with very poor recognition by the general practitioners; only 2 of 110 cases of ADs were identified clinically by them. A German study in community settings identified a prevalence of 0.9% when clinically significant impairment was a criterion; an additional 1.4% of subjects were diagnosed with ADs without meeting the impairment criterion (Maercker et al. 2007, 2012). A multicenter study found an AD prevalence rate of 1% (Ayuso-Mateos et al. 2001).

Andreasen and Wasek (1980) observed that 5% of inpatient and outpatient cohorts were diagnosed with ADs. Fabrega et al. (1987) noted that 2.3% of patients in a walk-in clinic (a diagnostic and evaluation center) met criteria for ADs with no other psychiatric diagnoses. When patients with other psychiatric diagnoses were included, 20% also had the diagnosis of an AD. In general hospital psychiatric consultation populations, ADs were diagnosed in 21.5% (Popkin et al. 1990), 18.5% (Oxman et al. 1994), and 11.5% (Snyder and Strain 1989) of patients. In palliative care a meta-analysis based on 24 studies identified ADs in 15.4% of subjects in comparison to a pooled prevalence of 14.3% for DSM-defined major depression and 16.5% for either DSM- or ICD-10-defined depressive disorder (Mitchell et al. 2011).

Strain et al. (1998) examined the consultation-liaison psychiatric data from seven university teaching hospitals in the United States, Canada, and Australia. The hospitals employed a common computerized clinical database to examine 1,039 consecutive psychiatric referrals—the MICRO-CARES software system. ADs were diagnosed in 125 patients (12.0%). They were the sole diagnosis in 81 (7.8%) and were comorbid with other psychiatric diagnoses in 44 (4.2%). They were considered a "rule-out" diagnosis in an additional 110 (10.6%). ADs with depressed mood, anxious mood, or mixed emotions were the most common subtypes. ADs were diagnosed comorbidly most frequently with personality disorder and organic mental disorder. Patients with ADs were referred for problems of anxiety, coping, and depression; had less past psychiatric illness; and were rated as previously functioning better than those patients with major mental disorders—all of which are consistent with the construct of ADs as a contemporary maladaptation to a stressor.

Psychiatric interventions in this inpatient cohort of consultation-liaison patients were similar to those used for other psychiatric diagnoses—in particular, the prescription of antidepressant medications. (This finding was in contrast to the consensus that the treatment of choice for ADs is psychotherapy and/or counseling, at least initially.) Patients with ADs required a similar amount of clinical treatment time and resident supervision time when compared with patients who had other psychiatric disorders (Strain et al. 1998).

Thus, ADs were not performing like a subthreshold (i.e., less serious) mental disorder in the psychiatric consultation setting with medically and surgically ill inpatients.

Oxman et al. (1994) reported that 50.7% of elderly patients (ages 55 years and older) receiving elective surgery for coronary artery disease developed ADs from the stress of surgery. Thirty percent had symptomatic and functional impairment 6 months after surgery. Kellermann et al. (1999) found that 27% of elderly patients examined 5–9 days after a cerebrovascular accident met the criteria for an AD. Spiegel (1996) reported that half of all cancer patients he studied had a psychiatric disorder, usually an AD with depression. ADs are frequently diagnosed in patients with head and neck cancer (16.8%; Kugaya et al. 2000), HIV (dementia and an AD) (73%; Pozzi et al. 1999), and cancer (from a multicenter survey of consultation-liaison psychiatry in oncology) (27%; Grassi et al. 2000); in dermatology inpatients (29% of the 9% who had psychiatric diagnoses; Pulimood et al. 1996); and in suicide attempters examined in an emergency department (22%; Schnyder and Valach 1997). ADs have also been diagnosed in more than 60% of burn inpatients (Perez Jimenez et al. 1994), 20% of patients in early stages of multiple sclerosis (Sullivan et al. 1995), and 40% of poststroke patients (Shima et al. 1994). Faulstich et al. (1986) reported a prevalence of 12.5% for DSM-III (American Psychiatric Association 1980) AD and conduct issues for adolescent psychiatric inpatients.

COURSE AND PROGNOSIS

The DSM-IV-TR Criterion E for ADs implies a good long-term outcome by stating that "once the stressor (or its consequences) has terminated, the symptoms do not persist for more than an additional 6 months" (American Psychiatric Association 2000, p. 683). Andreasen and Hoenk's (1982) landmark study supported the validity of this statement by showing that prognosis was favorable for adults; however, prognosis was less favorable for adolescents, many of whom developed major psychiatric illnesses over time. At 5-year follow-up, 71% of the adults were completely well, 8% had an intervening problem, and 21% had developed a major depressive disorder or alcoholism. Of the adolescents at 5-year follow-up, only 44% were without a psychiatric diagnosis, whereas 13% had experienced an intervening psychiatric illness and 43% had developed major psychiatric morbidity (e.g., schizophrenia, schizoaffective disorder, major depression, bipolar disorder, substance abuse, personality disorders). In contrast to the predictors for major pathology in adults, the chronicity of the illness and the presence of behavioral symptoms in the adolescents were the strongest predictors for major pathology at 5-year follow-up. As predictors of future outcome, the numbers and types of symptoms were less useful than the length of treatment and chronicity of symptoms.

ADs with disturbance of conduct, regardless of age, have a more guarded outcome. Just as Andreasen and Wasek (1980) observed, Chess and Thomas (1984) underscored that a significant number of patients with ADs either do not improve or grow worse in adolescence and early adult life. Kovacs et al. (1994) examined children and youth (ages 8–13 years) for up to 8 years and, controlling for the effects of comorbidity, observed that ADs do not predict later dysfunction. Jones et al. (2002) described 10 years of readmission data for various psychiatric diagnoses and observed that patients with ADs had the lowest readmission rates. Initial psychological recovery from an AD may be attributable to removal of the stressor or recovery from the effects of the stressor. This was the case in prisoners who developed ADs after being placed in solitary confinement and whose symptoms resolved shortly after their release (Andersen et al. 2000).

Supporting the clinical significance of ADs, Runeson et al. (1996) found that a shorter interval before suicidal behavior occurred following the diagnosis of ADs (1 month) than the diagnosis of depression (3 months), borderline personality disorder (30 months), or schizophrenia (47 months). Casey et al. (2015) identified self-harm as occurring at a lower symptom threshold in those with ADs than in those with ICD-10-defined depressive episode and with lower suicide intent scores in the objective circumstances measure. Portzky et al. (2005) conducted psychological autopsies on adolescents with ADs who had committed suicide and found that suicidal thinking in these patients was brief and evolved rapidly and without warning, complicating any attempt at timely intervention. Among adults in some cultures, ADs are the most common diagnosis in those dying by suicide (Manoranjitham et al. 2010); the diagnosis of ADs may be the only indicator of this life-threatening behavior.

A slightly different profile was found in two other studies that looked at suicide attempters with a diagnosis of an AD (Kryzhanovskaya and Canterbury 2001; Pelkonen et al. 2005). These patients were more likely to have comorbid personality disorders, poor overall psychosocial functioning, a history of prior psychiatric treatment, substance abuse histories, and a current "mixed" symptom profile of depressed mood and behavioral disturbances. Casey et al. (2015) examined the issue of suicidal ideation in a consultation-liaison cohort.

A study of the neurochemical variables of AD patients of all ages who had attempted suicide revealed biological correlates consistent with the more major psychiatric disorders (Lindqvist et al. 2008). Compared with control subjects, attempters exhibited lower platelet monoamine oxidase activity, higher 3-methoxy-4-hydroxyphenylglycol (MHPG) activity, and higher cortisol levels. Although these findings for patients with ADs differ from the lower MHPG and cortisol levels found in patients with major depression and suicidality, they are similar to the observations in other major stress-related conditions.

Despland et al. (1997) observed 52 patients with ADs at the end of treatment or after 3 years of treatment; results showed the occurrence of psychiatric comorbidity (31%), suicide attempts (14%), development of a more serious psychiatric disorder (29%), and an unfavorable clinical state (23%). Spalletta et al. (1996) stated that suicidal behavior and deliberate self-harm are important symptoms that forecast a possible diagnosis of an AD. Clearly, suicidal behavior by some patients with ADs indicates that ADs are *not* a subthreshold disorder in regard to their potential consequences.

DIAGNOSIS

Most individuals who are diagnosed with ADs have no prior psychiatric history. A close temporal relationship exists between a triggering event and AD symptom onset, and the symptoms may worsen when there is cognitive proximity to the stressor (e.g., while talking about it or when reexposed to the stressful situation, such as the resumption of symptoms when an individual who has been subjected to workplace bullying returns to work after being on sick leave).

For the differential diagnosis of ADs, the clinician needs to consider 1) no psychiatric diagnosis (i.e., normal stress reaction), 2) minor depressive disorder, 3) major depressive disorder, 4) anxiety disorder, 5) posttraumatic stress disorder and acute stress disorder, and 6) mood alteration secondary to substance abuse.

TREATMENT

Psychotherapy

Treatment of ADs relies primarily on psychotherapeutic measures that enable reduction of the stressor, enhanced coping with stressors that cannot be reduced or removed, and establishment of a support system to maximize adaptation. The first goal for the therapist is to note significant dysfunction secondary to a stressor and to help the patient moderate this imbalance. Many stressors (e.g., taking on more responsibility than can be managed by the individual or putting oneself at risk by having unprotected sex with an unknown partner) can be avoided or minimized. Other stressors (e.g., abandonment by a lover) may elicit an overreaction on the part of the patient. The patient may attempt suicide or become reclusive, damaging his or her source of income. In these situations, the therapist attempts to help the patient put his or her distress and other feelings into words rather than into destructive actions and to assist with more optimal adaptation to and mastery of the trauma or stressor. The role of verbalization cannot be overestimated as an effective approach to reducing the impact of the stressor and to enhance coping. The therapist needs to clarify and interpret the meaning of the stressor for the patient. For example, a mastectomy

may have devastated a patient's feelings about her body and herself. It is necessary to clarify that the patient is still a woman, capable of having a fulfilling relationship, including a sexual one, and that the patient can have the cancer
removed or treated and not necessarily have a recurrence. Otherwise, the patient's pernicious fantasies—"all is lost"—may take over in response to the
stressor (i.e., the mastectomy) and make her dysfunctional in work and/or relationships (including sex), precipitating a painful disturbance of mood that is in-
capacitating.

Counseling, psychotherapy, cognitive-behavioral therapy (CBT), interpersonal therapy, medical crisis counseling, crisis intervention, family therapy, and
supportive group treatment may be employed to encourage the verbalization of
fears, anxiety, rage, helplessness, and hopelessness related to the stressors imposed on (or self-imposed by) a patient. CBT was successfully used in young
military recruits (Nardi et al. 1994).

The goals of treatment in each case are to expose the concerns and conflicts
that the patient is experiencing, identify strategies to reduce the stressors, enhance
the patient's coping skills, help the patient gain perspective on the adversity, and
help the patient establish relationships (e.g., a support network) to assist in the
management of the stressors and the self.

Brief Psychotherapy

Sifneos (1989) stated that patients with ADs (diagnosed using DSM-III-R criteria [American Psychiatric Association 1987]) can profit most from brief psychotherapy. The psychotherapy should attempt to reframe the meaning of the
stressor(s). Although brief therapeutic interventions are often sufficient, ongoing stressors or enduring character pathology that may make a patient vulnerable to stress intolerance may signal the need for lengthier treatments.

Many types of therapeutic modalities have a place in the treatment of ADs.
Wise (1988), drawing from military psychiatry, emphasized the treatment variables of brevity, immediacy, centrality, expectance, proximity, and simplicity
(BICEPS principles) (Wise 1988). The treatment approach for BICEPS is brief,
usually not planned for all sessions to last more than 72 hours (True and Benway 1992).

Interpersonal Psychotherapy

Interpersonal psychotherapy was applied to depressed HIV-positive outpatients and was found to be effective (Markowitz et al. 1992). The mechanisms
of interpersonal psychotherapy are important in understanding psychotherapeutic approaches to the ADs: 1) psychoeducation about the sick role, 2) a here-
and-now framework, 3) formulation of the problems from an interpersonal
perspective, 4) exploration of options for changing dysfunctional behavior pat-

terns, 5) identification of focused interpersonal problem areas, and 6) the confidence that therapists gain from a systematic approach to problem formulation and treatment.

Psychotherapy for the Elderly

Elderly patients are particularly vulnerable to the development of ADs as a result of multiple stresses related to interpersonal losses, medical illnesses, and multiple medications. Life transitions such as relocating to a nursing home or losing one's driving privileges are commonly experienced as stressors by elderly individuals. Treatments that strengthen a patient's ego functions by helping him or her acknowledge the stressor and by promoting effective coping strategies are useful in this population. An active therapeutic stance and the use of life review foster a sense of mastery over the stressor (Frankel 2001).

Support Groups

Attending support groups helps patients with ADs adjust and enhances their coping mechanisms (Fawzy et al. 2003; Spiegel et al. 1989). Studies of the survival benefits of psychosocial group interventions have mixed results. Cancer patients who attended support groups have experienced increased survival time, improvements in mood, reduced distress level, and enhanced quality of life (Akechi et al. 2008; Goodwin et al. 2001; Newell et al. 2002; Spiegel 2011; Spiegel et al. 2007).

Eye Movement Desensitization

Eye movement desensitization and reprocessing, which is effective in the treatment of posttraumatic stress disorder, was used with nine patients with ADs (Mihelich 2000). Results demonstrated significant improvement among patients with anxious or mixed features but not among those with depressed mood. Also, those patients with ongoing stressors did not demonstrate improvement.

Occupational Intervention, Cognitive-Behavioral Approach, and Problem-Solving Treatment

The Cochrane database revealed only two randomized controlled trials (RCTs) of specific psychotherapeutic treatment of ADs. In one, Gonzalez-Jaimes and Turnbull-Plaza (2003) observed that mirror psychotherapy for AD patients with depressed mood secondary to a myocardial infarction was both an efficient and an effective treatment. Mirror therapy can be described as comprising psychocorporal, cognitive, and neurolinguistic components with a holistic focus. As part of the treatment, a mirror is used to encourage a patient's acceptance of his or her physical limitations that resulted from the lack of past self-care behaviors. Mirror therapy was compared with two other treatments—Gestalt psychotherapy and medical conversation—and a control condition. Depressive symptoms improved in all treatment groups compared with the control group, but mirror therapy was significantly more effective than other treatments in decreasing symptoms of ADs at posttest evaluation.

In another RCT, an "activating intervention" for ADs was employed for occupational dysfunction (van der Klink and van Dijk 2003). A total of 192 employees were randomly assigned to receive either the intervention or usual care. The intervention consisted of an individual cognitive-behavioral approach to a graded activity, similar to stress inoculation training. The worker was asked to do more demanding and complicated activities as treatment progressed. Goals of treatment emphasized the acquisition of coping skills and the regaining of control. The treatment proved to be effective in decreasing sick leave duration and shortening long-term absenteeism when compared with the control cohort. Both intervention and control groups, however, showed similar amounts of symptom reduction. This study formed the basis for the Dutch practice guidelines for treating ADs in primary and occupational health care (van der Klink et al. 2003); these guidelines were prepared by 21 occupational health physicians and one psychologist and subsequently were reviewed and tested by 15 experts, including several psychiatrists and psychologists and 21 practicing occupational health physicians.

In a Cochrane database review, Arends et al. (2012) evaluated 59 RCTs involving workplace interventions using CBT and problem-solving treatment for individuals with ADs and found only 9 to be scientifically adequate for inclusion in the meta-analysis. However, those 9 studies had the major problem of heterogeneity of psychiatric diagnosis. "Burnout," "stress," "neurasthenia," "work-related stress," and "minor mental disorder" were considered as diagnoses of ADs in several studies, which further dilutes the definition of this already problematically defined psychiatric disorder. Some studies were included if as few as 30% of the diagnoses were "pure" ADs. Finally, ADs were diagnosed using various criteria, screening instruments, and diagnosticians. The authors found that although problem-solving treatment was superior to no treatment, it did not reduce the number of days to either partial or full-time return to work when compared with no treatment. Compared with non-guideline-based care, however, problem-solving therapy did reduce the time to partial return to work but did not influence the number of days to full-time return.

Brief Dynamic and Brief Supportive Therapies

Although no other RCTs involving the psychotherapeutic treatment of pure cohorts of patients with ADs could be found, many exist that studied an array of depressive and anxiety disorders and included ADs in their cohorts. A trial comparing brief dynamic therapy with brief supportive therapy in treating patients with minor depressive disorders, including ADs (therefore a mixed diagnostic sample), was reported in the Cochrane database. Although both therapies proved efficacious in reducing symptoms, brief dynamic therapy was more effective at 6-month follow-up (Maina et al. 2005).

Akechi et al. (2008) investigated associated and predictive factors in cancer patients with ADs and major depression. Findings revealed that psychological distress in these patients was associated with a variety of factors, including reduced social support, impaired physical functioning, and existential concerns. This study highlights the necessity of a multidimensional care plan for the treatment of ADs that includes physical, psychosocial, and existential components. Studies have yet to evaluate the potential role of family and couples therapy as well as complementary alternative medicine such as acupuncture and yoga.

Pharmacotherapy

Although psychotherapy is the mainstay of treatment for ADs, Stewart et al. (1992) emphasized the importance of including psychopharmacological interventions in the treatment of minor depression. These authors argued that pharmacotherapy is generally recommended, but data do not support this contention. Despite the lack of rigorous scientific evidence, Stewart and colleagues advocated successive trials with antidepressants in any depressed patient (major or minor disorders), particularly if he or she has not benefited from psychotherapy or other supportive measures for 3 months. The authors did not mention ADs with depressed mood in particular. An RCT in the treatment of minor depressive disorder showed that fluoxetine proved superior to placebo in reducing depressive symptoms, improving overall psychosocial functioning, and alleviating suffering (Judd 2000). The question remains whether this also applies to ADs with depressed mood.

The following patient, diagnosed with an AD with depressed mood, did not respond to counseling and was sufficiently distressed by her mood disorder to require a pharmacotherapeutic intervention.

Case Vignette

Mrs. W, a 35-year-old married woman and mother of three children, was desperate when she learned that she had cancer and would need a mastectomy followed by chemotherapy and radiation. She was convinced that she would not recover, that her body would be forever distorted and ugly, that her husband would no longer find her attractive, and that her children would be ashamed of her baldness and the fact that she had cancer. She wondered if anyone would ever want to touch her again. Her mother and sister had also experienced breast cancer, and she felt that she was fated to have an empty future.

Despite several sessions to deal with her feelings, Mrs. W's dysphoria remained profound. She exhibited no vegetative signs indicating major depression, she was not anhedonic or guilt-ridden, and she admitted no suicidal ideation. She did not have two of the eight vegetative or ideational symptoms to qualify for DSM-IV-TR minor depressive disorder. Her clinician decided to add antidepressant pharmacotherapy (fluoxetine 20 mg/day) to her psychotherapy sessions to decrease her continuing unpleasant mood state. Two weeks later, Mrs. W reported that she was feeling less despondent and less concerned about the future. As she came to terms with the overwhelming stressor and was assisted with antidepressant agents, her depressed mood improved and her ability to employ more adequate coping strategies to handle her serious medical illness was mobilized.

RCTs of the use of pharmacotherapy in patients with ADs are rare. Formal psychotherapy appears to be the treatment of choice (Uhlenhuth et al. 1995), although psychotherapy combined with benzodiazepines also is used, especially for patients with severe life stress(ors) and a significant anxious component (Shaner 2000; Uhlenhuth et al. 1995). Tricyclic antidepressants or the anxiolytic buspirone are recommended in place of benzodiazepines for patients with current or past heavy alcohol use because of the greater risk of dependence (Uhlenhuth et al. 1995). In a 25-week multicenter RCT, a special extract from kava kava (WS 1490) was reported to be effective in treating ADs with anxiety, in comparison with placebo, and did not produce side effects, as is the case with tricyclics and benzodiazepines (Volz and Kieser 1997).

In an RCT, Bourin et al. (1997) assigned patients to receive either Euphytose—a preparation containing a combination of plant extracts (*Crataegus, Ballota, Passiflora,* and *Valeriana,* which have mild sedative effects, and *Cola* and *Paullinia,* which mainly act as mild stimulants)—or placebo. Patients taking the experimental drugs improved significantly more than those taking placebo. In another study, tianeptine, alprazolam, and mianserin were found to be equally effective in symptom improvement in patients with ADs with anxiety (Ansseau et al. 1996). In an RCT, trazodone was more effective than clorazepate in cancer patients for the relief of anxious and depressed symptoms (Razavi et al. 1999). Similar findings were observed in HIV-positive patients with ADs (DeWit et al. 1999).

There are no RCTs employing selective serotonin reuptake inhibitors (SSRIs), other antidepressants, or anxiolytics (e.g., nefazodone, venlafaxine, buspirone, mirtazapine). These medications may offer symptom relief of dysphoric or anxious moods. The difficulty in obtaining an AD study cohort with reliable and valid diagnoses may impede the ability to conduct an RCT comparing these agents against placebo and psychotherapy. The stressor attributes add a further confound to obtaining a homogeneous sample because of the differences in the stressors, including nature (quality), severity (quantity), and duration (acute vs. chronic).

Clinical trials regarding ADs are also compromised by patients' not having specific symptoms to monitor when examining the outcome of an intervention.

Timing and chronicity are other issues. In the case of the ADs, it is not known whether the therapeutic outcome should be assessed when the stressors have stabilized, when the stressors have abated, or after an agreed-on time period (e.g., 3 months) has elapsed.

Psychotropic medication has been used in medically ill patients, terminally ill patients, and patients with illness refractory to verbal therapies. Many of these patients had ADs, but it cannot be certain if some had minor depression. In a study of medically ill patients with unspecified depressive disorders (which may not have been ADs), Rosenberg et al. (1991) reported that 16 of 29 patients (55%) improved within 2 days of treatment with the maximal dosage of amphetamine derivatives. The presence of delirium was associated with a decreased response. Whether methylphenidate would be useful in ADs with depressed mood remains to be investigated, but this drug has the problem of potential for addiction.

In a review of RCTs, Reynolds (1992) stated that bereavement-related syndromal depression appears to respond to antidepressant medication. If medication is prescribed for minor disorders (including subthreshold disorders), the predominant mood that accompanies the (adjustment) disorder is an important consideration. Schatzberg (1990) recommended that therapists consider both psychotherapy and pharmacotherapy in ADs with anxious mood and that anxiolytics should be part of psychiatrists' armamentarium. Nguyen et al. (2006), using an RCT, compared the efficacies of etifoxine, a nonbenzodiazepine anxiolytic drug, and lorazepam, a benzodiazepine, in the treatment of ADs with anxiety in a primary care setting. Efficacy was evaluated on days 7 and 28 using the Hamilton Anxiety Rating Scale. The two drugs were found to be equivalent in anxiolytic efficacy on day 28. However, more etifoxine recipients responded to the treatment. One week after stopping treatment, fewer patients taking etifoxine experienced rebound anxiety compared with those on lorazepam.

Stein (2015) studied the effects of etifoxine versus alprazolam for the treatment of ADs with anxiety in an RCT. The findings provide support for the efficacy and safety of etifoxine in the management of ADs with anxiety, particularly when treatment discontinuation data are also assessed. Etifoxine has the important clinical advantage of having anxiolytic effects, which are not associated with dependence. Pharmacotherapy was equally efficacious in patients with more severe anxiety symptoms at baseline.

A new Cochrane meta-analysis is under way examining the psychopharmacological treatment of ADs. This is an important investigation because few RCTs of psychopharmacological treatment of ADs exist (Casey et al. 2013). Although the protocol has been published, results are not yet available.

Regardless of whether psychotherapy or pharmacotherapy is used alone or in combination, a significant aspect of treatment is to recognize that the diagnosis of an AD may indicate that a patient is in the early phase of a major mental disorder that has not yet evolved to full-blown symptoms. If the patient continues to worsen, becomes more symptomatic, and does not respond to treatment, it is critical to review the patient's symptom profile and consider whether the AD has progressed to a major mental disorder. Mrs. W, the patient in the earlier case vignette, may have been in the early phase of a major depressive disorder, but at the time of assessment, she met criteria only for an AD with depressed mood, a subthreshold mood disorder.

Resilience

In articles on the implications of resilience in the prevention and treatment of depression, Southwick and Charney (2012) and Southwick et al. (2014) expound on the need to better understand the psychobiology of resilience as an important component of effective treatment for stress-induced dysfunction and distress. The authors emphasize that persons react remarkably differently to stress, depending on numerous genetic, developmental, cognitive, psychological, and neurobiological risk and protective factors. The authors define their understanding of resilience as the ability to bounce back from hardship and trauma. The American Psychological Association defines resilience as the process of adapting well in the face of adversity, trauma, tragedy, threats, or significant sources of threat (Duman and Aghajanian 2012). Overwhelming stressors in childhood may lead to "giving in and giving up" to later stressors, whereas manageable stressors in childhood may actually strengthen the individual's capacity to cope with stress later on. This is an entirely different conceptual framework of systematizing the etiology of distress and dysfunction in ADs and also offers an alternative route to treatment. According to Southwick and Charney (2012), the development of therapeutic agents to contain excessive amounts of stress-induced corticotropin releasing hormone, which controls and integrates the body's response to stress, might reduce rates of trauma- and stressor-related psychopathology. (Resilience is discussed in more detail in Chapter 9, "Therapeutic Adaptations of Resilience.")

Treatment of ADs in Primary Care

It is important to note that the ADs involve various symptom types: depression, anxiety, conduct disturbance, and mixtures of these. Although what follows emphasizes depression, the other subtypes also need to be kept in mind as ideal candidates to be treated in the primary care setting—there are just less information and research regarding them. Furthermore, there is a lack of sufficient distinction between ADs with depression and the entity of minor depression (see Chapter 3, "Conceptual Framework and Controversies in Adjustment Disorders"). Primary care is an important venue for the identification and treatment of depression, including ADs. The Agency for Health Care Policy and Research (1993) developed guidelines for the treatment of depression in primary care but not specifically for ADs with depression. If any depressive disorder could be treated in primary care, ADs with depressed mood—too often regarded as a subthreshold disorder—would be the most likely candidate.

Although ADs were not the focus of the studies by Wayne Katon and his colleagues, their approach to bringing together the practices of primary care and psychiatry to treat patients with mental health issues could serve as a template for treating ADs as well. His group examined depression treatment issues in real-world settings, including the measurement of disability and cost; in addition, they addressed the issue of effectiveness research and its needed methodology (Katon 1999). Katon conducted an RCT at the University of Washington to determine the specificity and intensity of mental health training programs that are necessary to ensure the sufficient transfer of knowledge from psychiatrists to primary care physicians for the identification and treatment of depressive disorders (Katon and Gonzales 1994). (Again, although this trial did not specifically identify ADs with depression as part of the study cohort, the procedure employed for knowledge transfer might apply to the AD subtypes as well.) This trial included providing education to the patient and the physician, as well as changing the structure of medical care delivery to enhance the primary care physician's capacity to adequately diagnose and treat depressive disorders. In an editorial on the "White Papers," a series of articles commissioned by the Services Research and Clinical Epidemiology Branch of the National Institute of Mental Health (NIMH) for the July 2000 NIMH Conference on Mental Health Services Research, Katon and Gonzales (2002) reported that

> programs aimed at physician education have had no lasting effects on patient outcomes, whereas *multimodal collaborative* intervention programs that integrated a range of physician extenders such as nurses or mental health specialists to increase rates of frequency of follow-up, monitor outcomes, activate patients to become partners in their care and facilitate referral to specialists have had marked effects on improving outcomes of depression for primary care patients. (p. 196)

Data indicate that informing the primary care physician that the patient has depression is not sufficient for enhancing patient outcome. Optimal therapeutic outcome in the primary care setting depends on three components: 1) sufficient patient education, 2) conjoint sessions with the psychiatrist and the primary care physician, and 3) sufficient follow-up by the psychiatrist during the course of treatment.

Barrett et al. (1999) undertook a comparison of paroxetine, problem-solving therapy, and placebo for minor depression and dysthymia in primary care patients. (ADs were not mentioned as included in the study cohort, so findings do not apply to the AD category.)

Strain et al. (1998) observed in multiple hospitals that patients with ADs seen in psychiatric consultation in the general hospital setting required as much of the psychiatric consultant's time and were just as likely to receive medication as were patients with major psychiatric disorders. As mentioned earlier in this section on treatment, ADs are currently thought to require talking treatment (psychotherapy and/or counseling), which takes time and is poorly reimbursed for primary care physicians. Because effective talking may require more skill than prescribing drugs, the possibility for treatment of pure ADs with depression, anxiety, conduct disturbance, or mixed symptoms in the primary care setting remains to be rigorously examined. However, the availability of multiple mental health practitioners and integrated mental health models of care, where care is delivered by mental health professionals who are embedded within the primary care practice, may offer an unprecedented opportunity for the treatment of the cadre of ADs.

Hameed et al. (2005), in a retrospective chart review, sought to determine whether there was a difference in antidepressant efficacy in the treatment of major depressive disorder versus ADs in a primary care setting. Patients had been prescribed mostly SSRIs. DSM-IV-TR symptoms, the Patient Health Questionnaire–9, depression rating scale scores, and functional disability reports were systematically used to assess patients' responses. Results showed that neither depressed patients nor patients with ADs demonstrated a difference in clinical response to any particular antidepressant. Patients with a diagnosis of an AD, however, were twice as likely as patients with major depression to respond to standard antidepressant treatment. This study suggests that antidepressants are effective in treating depression in the primary care setting and may be even more effective in the treatment for ADs with depressed mood. Companion studies examining anxiolytics and their outcome in ADs with anxiety are warranted.

FUTURE DIRECTIONS

Understanding of the etiology of depression and its treatment has advanced with discoveries about the neurobiology of affective disorders and the utilization of animal models (Friedman et al. 2011). The neurobiology of major disorders, including the anxiety disorders, may offer new pathways for the minor, subsyndromal diagnoses, such as ADs with anxiety. Duman and Aghajanian (2012) presented their hypothesis that synaptic dysfunction causes depression and proposed potential therapeutic targets. They discussed that ketamine, an N-methyl-D-aspartate receptor antagonist, has been found to produce rapid antidepressant responses in treatment-resistant patients with depression. Ketamine induces synaptogenesis and reverses the synaptic deficits caused by chronic stress, including neuronal atrophy and decreases in synaptic density (synaptic loss). A relevant study for ADs would be whether this mechanism of therapeutic action would have any effect on ADs with depressed mood, especially the chronic form. This possibility again emphasizes the value of understanding the relationship, if any, between subsyndromal symptoms and fully developed symptom profiles of the major syndromes. This would enhance our understanding of the treatment regimens that may aptly be utilized with the ADs.

CONCLUSION

The ADs are the most common diagnoses in military personnel, in children, and in psychosomatic medicine or consultation-liaison psychiatry settings. There are few outcome studies regarding the current interventions. It is not known what percentage of people with ADs experience spontaneous recovery, progress to major disorder symptomatology, or retain a chronic form of subsyndromal AD. It is essential to learn more about diagnosing this common mental disorder, as well as the interventions most likely to have a salutary response and in what setting (e.g., integrated primary care health settings) these interventions are most effective. Current and future neuroscience breakthroughs may open a pathway to a more rigorous understanding of these ubiquitous disorders.

Key Points

- Psychotherapies are a first line of treatment for the adjustment disorders (ADs).

- Reduction of the stressor and its effects are important targets of the therapeutic intervention.

- ADs are common diagnoses among military personnel, children, and medically ill patients.

- The diagnosis of ADs in children and youth is a risk factor for the later development of more serious psychiatric disorders.

- Suicide often occurs in patients with the diagnosis of ADs.

- Psychotherapies for treatment include brief psychotherapy, interpersonal psychotherapy, occupational problem-solving treatment, brief dynamic therapy, and brief supportive therapy.

- Elderly individuals are particularly vulnerable to developing AD.

- Pharmacotherapies can be employed according to the AD's concomitant mood (e.g., depression, anxiety).

- Few randomized controlled trials have been done involving selective serotonin reuptake inhibitors or anxiolytics in treating ADs.

- Treatment of the ADs in primary care is compromised by time constraints that affect the physician's ability to offer time-consuming talking interventions.

SUGGESTED READINGS

Casey P: Adjustment disorder: epidemiology, diagnosis and treatment. CNS Drugs 23(11):927–938, 2009 19845414

Strain JJ, Friedman MJ: Considering adjustment disorders as stress response syndromes for DSM-5. Depress Anxiety 28(9):818–823, 2011 21254314

REFERENCES

Agency for Health Care Policy and Research: Depression Guideline Panel: Depression in Primary Care, Vol 1: Diagnosis and Detection; Vol 2: Treatment of Major Depression. Clinical Practice Guideline No 5 (AHCPR Publ No 93-0550, 93-0551). Rockville, MD, U.S. Department of Health and Human Services, Public Health Service, Agency for Health Care Policy and Research, 1993

Akechi T, Okuyama T, Onishi J, et al: Psychotherapy for depression among incurable cancer patients. Cochrane Database Syst Rev (2):CD005537, 2008 18425922

American Psychiatric Association: Diagnostic and Statistical Manual of Mental Disorders, 3rd Edition. Washington, DC, American Psychiatric Association, 1980

American Psychiatric Association: Diagnostic and Statistical Manual of Mental Disorders, 3rd Edition, Revised. Washington, DC, American Psychiatric Association, 1987

American Psychiatric Association: Diagnostic and Statistical Manual of Mental Disorders, 4th Edition. Washington, DC, American Psychiatric Association, 1994

American Psychiatric Association: Diagnostic and Statistical Manual of Mental Disorders, 4th Edition, Text Revision. Washington, DC, American Psychiatric Association, 2000

Andersen HS, Sestoft D, Lillebaek T, et al: A longitudinal study of prisoners on remand: psychiatric prevalence, incidence and psychopathology in solitary vs. non-solitary confinement. Acta Psychiatr Scand 102(1):19–25, 2000 10892605

Andreasen NC, Hoenk PR: The predictive value of adjustment disorders: a follow-up study. Am J Psychiatry 139:584–590, 1982 7072842

Andreasen NC, Wasek P: Adjustment disorders in adolescents and adults. Arch Gen Psychiatry 37:1166–1170, 1980 7425801

Ansseau M, Bataille M, Briole G, et al: Controlled comparison of tianeptine, alprazolam and mianserin in the treatment of ADs with anxiety and depression. Hum Psychopharmacol 11:293–298, 1996

Arends I, Bruinvels DJ, Rebergen DS, et al: Interventions to facilitate return to work in adults with adjustment disorders. Cochrane Database Syst Rev (12):CD006389, 2012 23235630

Ayuso-Mateos JL, Vázquez-Barquero JL, Dowrick C, et al; ODIN Group: Depressive disorders in Europe: prevalence figures from the ODIN study. Br J Psychiatry 179:308–316, 2001 11581110

Barrett JE, Williams JW Jr, Oxman TE, et al: The treatment effectiveness project. A comparison of the effectiveness of paroxetine, problem-solving therapy, and placebo in the treatment of minor depression and dysthymia in primary care patients: background and research plan. Gen Hosp Psychiatry 21(4):260–273, 1999 10514950

Bourin M, Bougerol T, Guitton B, et al: A combination of plant extracts in the treatment of outpatients with adjustment disorder with anxious mood: controlled study versus placebo. Fundam Clin Pharmacol 11:127–132, 1997 9107558

Brezinka C, Huter O, Biebl W, et al: Denial of pregnancy: obstetrical aspects. J Psychosom Obstet Gynaecol 15(1):1–8, 1994 8038884

Casey P, Pillay D, Wilson L, et al: Pharmacological interventions for adjustment disorders in adults (protocol). Cochrane Database Syst Rev (6):CD010530, 2013

Casey P, Jabbar F, O'Leary E, et al: Suicidal behaviours in adjustment disorder and depressive episode. J Affect Disord 174:441–446, 2015 25553405

Chess S, Thomas A: Origins and Evolution of Behavior Disorders: From Infancy to Early Adult Life. New York, Brunner/Mazel, 1984

Cohen F: Stress and bodily illness. Psychiatr Clin North Am 4(2):269–286, 1981 7024936

Despland JN, Monod L, Ferrero F: Etude clinique du trouble de l'adaptation selon le DSM-III-R. Schweiz Arch Neurol Neurochir Psychiatr 148:19–24, 1997

DeWit S, Cremers L, Hirsch D, et al: Efficacy and safety of trazodone versus clorazepate in the treatment of HIV-positive subjects with adjustment disorders: a pilot study. J Int Med Res 27:223–232, 1999 10689628

Duman RS, Aghajanian GK: Synaptic dysfunction in depression: potential therapeutic targets. Science 338(6103):68–72, 2012 23042884

Fabrega HJr, Mezzich JE, Mezzich AC: Adjustment disorder as a marginal or transitional illness category in DSM-III. Arch Gen Psychiatry 44:567–572, 1987 3579503

Faulstich ME, Moore JR, Carey MP, et al: Prevalence of DSM-III conduct and adjustment disorder for adolescent psychiatric inpatients. Adolescence 21(82):333–337, 1986 3739828

Fawzy FI, Canada AL, Fawzy NW: Malignant melanoma: effects of a brief, structured psychiatric intervention on survival and recurrence at 10-year follow-up. Arch Gen Psychiatry 60(1):100–103, 2003 12511177

Fernández A, Mendive JM, Salvador-Carulla L, et al: Adjustment disorders in primary care: prevalence, recognition and use of services. Br J Psychiatry 201:137–142, 2012 22576725

For-Wey L, Fei-Yin L, Bih-Ching S: The relationship between life adjustment and parental bonding in military personnel with adjustment disorder in Taiwan. Mil Med 167:678–682, 2002 12188241

Frankel M: Ego enhancing treatment of adjustment disorders of later life. J Geriatr Psychiatry 34:221–223, 2001

Friedman MJ, Resick PA, Bryant RA, et al: Classification of trauma and stressor-related disorders in DSM-5. Depress Anxiety 28(9):737–749, 2011 21681870

Giotakos O, Konstantakopoulos G: Parenting received in childhood and early separation anxiety in male conscripts with adjustment disorder. Mil Med 167(1):28–33, 2002 11799809

Gonzalez-Jaimes EI, Turnbull-Plaza B: Selection of psychotherapeutic treatment for adjustment disorder with depressive mood due to acute myocardial infarction. Arch Med Res 34:298–304, 2003 12957527

Goodwin PJ, Leszcz M, Ennis M, et al: The effect of group psychosocial support on survival in metastatic breast cancer. N Engl J Med 345(24):1719–1726, 2001 11742045

Grassi L, Gritti P, Rigatelli M, Gala C; Italian Consultation-Liaison Group: Psychosocial problems secondary to cancer: an Italian multicentre survey of consultation-liaison psychiatry in oncology. Eur J Cancer 36(5):579–585, 2000 10738121

Hameed U, Schwartz TL, Malhotra K, et al: Antidepressant treatment in the primary care office: outcomes for adjustment disorder versus major depression. Ann Clin Psychiatry 17:77–81, 2005 16075660

Jones R, Yates WR, Zhou MD: Readmission rates for adjustment disorders: comparison with other mood disorders. J Affect Disord 71:199–203, 2002 12167517

Judd LL: Diagnosis and treatment of minor depressive disorders. Int J Neuropsychopharmacol 3(suppl):S66, 2000

Katon W: Treatment trials in real world settings. Methodological issues and measurement of disability and costs. Gen Hosp Psychiatry 21(4):237–238, 1999 10514946

Katon W, Gonzales J: A review of randomized trials of psychiatric consultation-liaison studies in primary care. Psychosomatics 35(3):268–278, 1994 8036256

Katon W, Gonzales J: Primary care and treatment of depression: a response to the NIMH "White Papers." Gen Hosp Psychiatry 24(4):194–196, 2002 12100829

Kellermann M, Fekete I, Gesztelyi R, et al: Screening for depressive symptoms in the acute phase of stroke. Gen Hosp Psychiatry 21(2):116–121, 1999 10228892

Kovacs M, Gatsonis C, Pollock M, et al: A controlled prospective study of DSM-III adjustment disorder in childhood. Short-term prognosis and long-term predictive validity. Arch Gen Psychiatry 51:535–541, 1994 8031226

Kryzhanovskaya L, Canterbury R: Suicidal behavior in patients with adjustment disorders. Crisis 22(3):125–131, 2001 11831599

Kugaya A, Akechi T, Okuyama T, et al: Prevalence, predictive factors, and screening for psychologic distress in patients with newly diagnosed head and neck cancer. Cancer 88(12):2817–2823, 2000 10870066

Lindqvist D, Traskman-Bendzl L, Vang F, et al: Suicidal intent and the HPA-axis characteristics of suicide attempters with major depression and adjustment disorders. Arch Suicide Res 12(3):197–207, 2008 18576201

Maercker A, Einsle F, Kollner V: Adjustment disorders as stress response syndromes: a new diagnostic concept and its exploration in a medical sample. Psychopathology 40(3):135–146, 2007 17284941

Maercker A, Forstmeier S, Pielmaier L, et al: Adjustment disorders: prevalence in a representative nationwide survey in Germany. Soc Psychiatry Psychiatr Epidemiol 47(11):1745–1752, 2012 22407021

Maina G, Forner F, Bogetto F: Randomized controlled trial comparing brief dynamic and supportive therapy with waiting list condition in minor depressive disorders. Psychother Psychosom 74(1):43–50, 2005 15627856

Manoranjitham SD, Rajkumar AP, Thangadurai P, et al: Risk factors for suicide in rural south India. Br J Psychiatry 196(1):26–30, 2010 20044655

Markowitz JC, Klerman GL, Perry SW: Interpersonal psychotherapy of depressed HIV-positive outpatients. Hosp Community Psychiatry 43(9):885–890, 1992 1427695

Mihelich ML: Eye movement desensitization and reprocessing treatment of adjustment disorder. Dissertation Abstracts International: Section B: The Sciences and Engineering 61:1091, 2000

Mitchell AJ, Chan M, Bhatti H, et al: Prevalence of depression, anxiety, and adjustment disorder in oncological, haematological, and palliative-care settings: a meta-analysis of 94 interview-based studies. Lancet Oncol 12:160–174, 2011 21251875

Nardi C, Lichtenberg P, Kaplan Z: Adjustment disorder of conscripts as a military phobia. Mil Med 159:612–616, 1994 7800178

Newell SA, Sanson-Fisher RW, Savolainen NJ: Systematic review of psychological therapies for cancer patients: overview and recommendations for future research. J Natl Cancer Inst 94(8):558–584, 2002

Nguyen N, Fakra E, Pradel V, et al: Efficacy of etifoxine compared to lorazepam monotherapy in the treatment of patients with adjustment disorders with anxiety: a double-blind controlled study in general practice. Hum Psychopharmacol 21:139–149, 2006 16625522

Oxman TE, Barrett JE, Freeman DH, et al: Frequency and correlates of adjustment disorder related to cardiac surgery in older patients. Psychosomatics 35:557–568, 1994 7809358

Pelkonen M, Marttunen M, Henriksson M, et al: Suicidality in adjustment disorder, clinical characteristics of adolescent outpatients. Eur Child Adolesc Psychiatry 14:174–180, 2005 15959663

Perez Jimenez JP, Gomez Bajo GJ, Lopez Castillo JJ, et al: Psychiatric consultation and post-traumatic stress disorder in burned patients. Burns 20(6):532–536, 1994 7880420

Popkin MK, Callies AL, Colon EA, et al: Adjustment disorder in medically ill patients referred for consultation in a university hospital. Psychosomatics 31:410–414, 1990 2247569

Portzky G, Audenaert K, van Heeringen K: Adjustment disorder and the course of the suicidal process in adolescents. J Affect Disord 87:265–270, 2005 16005078

Pozzi G, Del Borgo C, Del Forno A, et al: Psychological discomfort and mental illness in patients with AIDS: implications for home care. AIDS Patient Care STDS 13(9):555–564, 1999 10813035

Pulimood S, Rajagopalan B, Rajagopalan M, et al: Psychiatric morbidity among dermatology inpatients. Natl Med J India 9(5):208–210, 1996 8937057

Razavi D, Kormoss N, Collard A, et al: Comparative study of the efficacy and safety of trazodone versus clorazepate in the treatment of adjustment disorders in cancer patients: a pilot study. J Int Med Res 27:264–272, 1999 10726235

Reynolds CF III: Treatment of depression in special populations. J Clin Psychiatry 53(suppl):45–53, 1992

Rosenberg PB, Ahmed I, Hurwitz S: Methylphenidate in depressed medically ill patients. J Clin Psychiatry 52(6):263–267, 1991 2055899

Runeson BS, Beskow J, Waern M: The suicidal process in suicides among young people. Acta Psychiatr Scand 93(1):35–42, 1996 8919327

Schatzberg AF: Anxiety and adjustment disorder: a treatment approach. J Clin Psychiatry 51(suppl):20–24, 1990 2228990

Schnyder U, Valach L: Suicide attempters in a psychiatric emergency room population. Gen Hosp Psychiatry 19(2):119–129, 1997 9097066

Shaner R: Benzodiazepines in psychiatric emergency settings. Psychiatr Ann 30:268–275, 2000

Shima S, Kitagawa Y, Kitamura T, et al: Poststroke depression. Gen Hosp Psychiatry 16(4):286–289, 1994 7926705

Sifneos PE: Brief dynamic and crisis therapy, in Comprehensive Textbook of Psychiatry IV, 5th Edition, Vol 2. Edited by Kaplan HI, Sadock BJ. Baltimore, MD, Williams & Wilkins, 1989, pp 1562–1567

Snyder S, Strain JJ: Differentiation of major depression and adjustment disorder with depressed mood in the medical setting. Gen Hosp Psychiatry 12:159–165, 1989 2335301

Southwick SM, Charney DS: The science of resilience: implications for the prevention and treatment of depression. Science 338(6103):79–82, 2012 23042887

Southwick MK, Bonanno GA, Masten AS, et al: Resilience definitions, theory, and challenges: interdisciplinary perspectives. Eur J Psychotraumatol 5, DOI: 10.3402/3jpt.v5.25338, 2014 [Epub] 25317257

Spalletta G, Troisi A, Saracco M, et al: Symptom profile, Axis II comorbidity and suicidal behaviour in young males with DSM-III-R depressive illnesses. J Affect Disord 39(2):141–148, 1996 8827424

Spiegel D: Cancer and depression. Br J Psychiatry Suppl 168(30)(suppl):109–116, 1996 8864156

Spiegel D: Mind matters in cancer survival. JAMA 305(5):502–503, 2011 21285429

Spiegel D, Bloom JR, Kraemer HC, et al: Effect of psychosocial treatment on survival of patients with metastatic breast cancer. Lancet 2(8668):888–891, 1989 2571815

Spiegel D, Butler LD, Giese-Davis J, et al: Effects of supportive-expressive group therapy on survival of patients with metastatic breast cancer: a randomized prospective trial. Cancer 110(5):1130–1138, 2007 17647221

Stein DJ: Etifoxine versus alprazolam for the treatment of adjustment disorder with anxiety: a randomized controlled trial. Adv Ther 32(1):57–68, 2015 25620535

Stewart JW, Quitkin FM, Klein DF: The pharmacotherapy of minor depression. Am J Psychother 46(1):23–36, 1992 1543251

Strain JJ, Smith GC, Hammer JS, et al: Adjustment disorder: a multisite study of its utilization and interventions in the consultation-liaison psychiatry setting. Gen Hosp Psychiatry 20:139–149, 1998 9650031

Sullivan MJ, Weinshenker B, Mikail S, et al: Screening for major depression in the early stages of multiple sclerosis. Can J Neurol Sci 22(3):228–231, 1995 8529176

True PK, Benway MW: Treatment of stress reaction prior to combat using the "BICEPS" model. Mil Med 157(7):380–381, 1992 1528476

Uhlenhuth EH, Balter MB, Ban TA, et al: International study of expert judgment on therapeutic use of benzodiazepines and other psychotherapeutic medications: III. Clinical features affecting experts' therapeutic recommendations in anxiety disorders. Psychopharmacol Bull 31(2):289–296, 1995 7491381

van der Klink JJ, van Dijk FJ: Dutch practice guidelines for managing adjustment disorders in occupational and primary health care. Scand J Work Environ Health 29:478–487, 2003 14712856

van der Klink JJ, Blonk RW, Schene AH, et al: Reducing long term sickness absence by an activating intervention in adjustment disorders: a cluster randomized controlled design. Occup Environ Med 60:429–437, 2003 12771395

Volz HP, Kieser M: Kava-kava extract WS 1490 versus placebo in anxiety disorders—a randomized placebo-controlled 25-week outpatient trial. Pharmacopsychiatry 30(1):1–5, 1997 9065962

Wise MG: Adjustment disorders and impulse disorders not otherwise classified, in American Psychiatric Press Textbook of Psychiatry. Edited by Talbot JA, Hales RE, Yudofsky SC. Washington, DC, American Psychiatric Press, 1988, pp 605–620

CHAPTER 5

Acute Stress Disorder

Richard A. Bryant, Ph.D.

THE DIAGNOSIS of acute stress disorder (ASD) has been surrounded by controversy since it was introduced. In this chapter I provide an overview of the diagnosis by reviewing the rationale for its introduction as a diagnosis, its definitions in DSM-IV (American Psychiatric Association 1994) and DSM-5 (American Psychiatric Association 2013), the evidence supporting its rationale, and treatment options available for managing people with ASD. The overarching theme of this chapter is that although ASD has been a "troubled" diagnosis since its inception, it has undoubtedly sparked much research, which has led to numerous theoretical and practical advances in how we understand and assist people with severe acute posttraumatic stress.

INTRODUCTION OF THE ACUTE STRESS DISORDER DIAGNOSIS

ASD was initially introduced for two reasons. The first was to account for severe acute stress reactions that occur in the initial month after a trauma. This goal arose because DSM has traditionally precluded posttraumatic stress disorder (PTSD) from being diagnosed until a month has elapsed after the trauma to minimize the likelihood of overpathologizing transient stress reactions. This wait time led to a situation in which clinicians were concerned that there was a "diagnostic gap" during which acutely traumatized people suffering marked distress could not be diagnosed. In some health care systems, particularly in the United States, this lack of diagnosis can hinder access to mental health care. To remedy this situation, clinicians argued that a diagnosis describing acute stress reactions would facilitate pathways to health care within a month of trauma exposure.

A second reason for the ASD diagnosis was to identify acutely traumatized people who are not experiencing a transient stress reaction but rather will subsequently develop PTSD. Clinicians argued that by introducing a diagnosis that differentiated those who had transient stress responses from those with the early stages of chronic posttraumatic stress, early intervention could be provided to limit development of PTSD.

ACUTE STRESS DISORDER IN DSM-IV

According to DSM-IV criteria for ASD, the individual had to be exposed to a traumatic event in which there was actual or threatened death or serious injury and to have experienced fear, helplessness, or horror (Criterion A). If the person satisfied this criterion, he or she was required to also meet four additional symptom clusters. Criterion B required at least three of the following dissociative symptoms: 1) a subjective sense of numbing, detachment, or absence of emotional responsiveness; 2) reduced awareness of surroundings; 3) derealization; 4) depersonalization; and 5) dissociative amnesia. These symptoms needed to exist either at the time of trauma or in the month afterward. The person also needed to exhibit one or more reexperiencing symptoms such as intrusive thoughts, images, nightmares, or distress at reminders of the event (Criterion C); marked avoidance of stimuli that remind the individual of the trauma (Criterion D); and marked anxiety or arousal symptoms (Criterion E). These symptoms had to cause significant distress or impairment (Criterion F) and last for a minimum of 2 days and a maximum of 4 weeks (Criterion G).

Apart from having different time frames, the main conceptual and operational difference between ASD and PTSD in DSM-IV was the emphasis placed on dissociative symptoms in ASD. It is useful to understand the reason behind this emphasis on dissociation. The historical roots of the role of dissociation could be traced back to the work of Pierre Janet in the early twentieth century. He argued that traumatized people may attempt to cope with intolerable experiences by splitting awareness of their distressed state from normal consciousness. According to this perspective, although this splitting resulted in some short-term relief, it nonetheless led to impaired mental health because of the demands placed on psychological resources. Interestingly, this perspective did not have great influence for much of the twentieth century, probably because of the dominance of psychoanalysis and the emerging influence of behaviorism. The view that dissociation is a pivotal factor in trauma response had a resurgence in the years before DSM-IV, which led some figures to argue that it needed a central role in diagnostic classification. In terms of ASD, it was argued that people who responded to a trauma with dissociative responses would be less able to access trauma memories and emotions, which would impede resolution of the experience and lead to ongoing PTSD (Spiegel et al. 1994). Consistent with this proposal, many studies have reported a relationship between acute dissociative responses and subsequent PTSD (Ehlers et al. 1998; Murray et al. 2002).

CONTROVERSIES ABOUT ACUTE STRESS DISORDER

Unlike most diagnoses, the ASD diagnosis met with considerable skepticism when it was introduced. The criticisms included both theoretical and empirical concerns. First, the idea that a major goal of ASD was to predict another subsequent, and phenomenologically similar, diagnosis was highly unusual and was criticized for confusing risk factors with diagnosis (Bryant and Harvey 2000). Second, at the time the diagnosis was introduced, there was a lack of evidence to support the new diagnosis (Bryant and Panasetis 2001). Even the proponents of the introduction of ASD acknowledged that the relationship between ASD and PTSD was "based more on logical arguments than on empirical research" (Koopman et al. 1995, p. 38). Third, there was concern that insufficient evidence existed to warrant the central role given to dissociative responses (Bryant and Panasetis 2001; Marshall et al. 1999). Fourth, because most people experience temporary distress after trauma exposure, there were concerns that the ASD diagnosis may lead to overpathologizing transient responses (Bryant and Harvey 2000; Marshall et al. 1999).

Not surprisingly, defendants of the new diagnosis responded to these criticisms. They emphasized that the limited evidence for the predictive ability of ASD to identify people who would develop PTSD should not be a critical concern because this was a secondary goal of ASD. They stressed that the primary aim of the ASD diagnosis is to identify severely distressed people who require mental health intervention but who would not be detected within the initial month (Simeon and Guralnik 2000). They also argued that the criticisms of the predictive power of ASD were unfair because the reason that ASD, and dissociative symptoms in particular, did not predict PTSD optimally was that dissociative symptoms were underrepresented in PTSD. Using a somewhat circular argument, they proposed that if the diagnosis of PTSD is amended to include more dissociative symptoms, then ASD would enjoy stronger predictive ability (Spiegel et al. 2000).

The diagnosis of ASD in DSM-IV also caused specific problems for clinicians insofar as its wording led to much ambiguity as to how one should interpret acute stress responses. The dissociative symptoms could be experienced either during or after the distressing event. At a mechanistic level, this vague time frame led to a situation in which if the dissociation occurs only during the event, then the alterations in perception and attention impede encoding of the experience. In contrast, if there is evidence of dissociation persisting in the weeks after the event, it is likely that it is impacting retrieval of the traumatic experience. Whereas the former scenario could be regarded as somewhat protective because it limited the amount of traumatic experience encoded, the latter could lead to psychopathology because it may impede resolution of the fear memories. Exemplifying this distinction is much evidence demonstrating that altered perceptions are very common under conditions of high stress—and indeed that they are experienced by most people. The following account of someone who was hit by a car on a road crossing illustrates this point.

> I remember hearing brakes screeching. I looked up and saw this car coming toward me. The brakes were slammed on, but it was skidding. Right at me. It was weird because it seemed to take forever to move. Like time stood still. I kept staring right at the car. In fact, I could not even tell you what my friends were doing next to me. They told me later they were yelling at me to run, but I never heard that. I just saw the car moving in slow motion toward me. But it all seemed so unreal.

This narrative includes a number of dissociative experiences listed in the DSM-IV criteria for ASD. The time slowing is a common example of derealization, in which one's surroundings seem to be dreamlike. Not hearing the friends yelling reflects reduced awareness of one's surroundings, and the inability to recall what they said could be interpreted as dissociative amnesia. All these responses are common in people who experience trauma and other high-stress situations, but they do not necessarily reflect the precursor of psychopathology. Supporting this perspective, studies that have assessed both peritraumatic and persistent dissociation have found that it is the dissociation that persists after exposure to the trauma that is linked to chronic (Briere et al. 2005) posttraumatic reactions.

It is also worth noting that the ASD criteria in DSM-IV were poorly articulated. Both the avoidance and arousal clusters required that "marked" levels of these symptoms be present for these clusters to be satisfied. Both of these reactions are very common after trauma; therefore, accurately assessing these symptoms when the only definition is that they are "marked" is problematic. The DSM-IV PTSD criteria had much clearer specification in terms of the number of symptoms required for each cluster (one for reexperiencing, three for avoidance, and two for arousal). Many clinicians were left wondering what the distinction was between normal and abnormal avoidance or arousal.

THE PREDICTIVE POWER OF ACUTE STRESS DISORDER

As noted in the first section of this chapter, one of the goals of the ASD diagnosis in DSM-IV was to identify acutely traumatized people who would subsequently develop PTSD. To test the predictive power of ASD, numerous studies were undertaken that assessed ASD in the initial month and later assessed the same people at varying times to establish their PTSD status. A systematic review of these studies identified 22 studies (4 with child populations) that used longitudinal designs to clarify the predictive capacity of ASD (Bryant 2011). One of the first points to emerge from these studies was that the positive predictive power of ASD in studies of adults was quite good; across most studies at least half of those trauma survivors who initially had ASD subsequently developed PTSD. This finding needs to be considered in light of the fact that most longitudinal studies indicate that most trauma survivors who are distressed in the initial period after trauma adapt in the following 6 months after exposure (Bryant 2003). The finding that people who meet criteria for ASD are generally at higher risk for PTSD supports the goal of predicting subsequent disorder.

The story was not so positive, however, regarding the sensitivity of these studies in predicting PTSD; that is, most trauma survivors who developed PTSD did not initially meet criteria for ASD. This finding suggests that the ASD diagnosis was failing in its goal of predicting PTSD. One reason put forward for this was the requirement that patients needed to satisfy the dissociative criterion. However, when considering the predictive capacity of subsyndromal ASD (which usually involved not requiring the dissociative criterion to be met), the sensitivity improved somewhat. In other words, when the focus was on general posttraumatic stress symptoms rather than the more restrictive requirement of dissociation, more people who developed PTSD were identified. However, even this strategy was very limited because it still resulted in a minority of people who developed PTSD being identified in the acute phase.

In terms of judging how well the ASD diagnosis can predict subsequent PTSD, it is worth noting that a lot more is now known about the course of posttraumatic adjustment. Put simply, PTSD does not follow a linear course. Instead, it fluctuates enormously in the months and years after trauma exposure. In one major longitudinal study, even though the rates of PTSD remained stable over the initial years after trauma exposure, only half of people who had PTSD at any assessment had the diagnosis at the following assessment (Bryant et al. 2013). This raises challenges for prediction of PTSD because it appears that a major reason the course of PTSD fluctuates over time is the occurrence of life stressors after the trauma. Therefore, the initial symptoms in the month after trauma can be expected to predict only a limited extent of subsequent PTSD, so prediction will always be modest.

ACUTE STRESS DISORDER AND RELATED DISORDERS

One of the major distinctions to make in differential diagnosis in the initial month after trauma is between ASD and adjustment disorder (AD). Like ASD,

AD can be diagnosed very shortly after exposure to an adverse situational event, but there are important differences. Most importantly, AD can be diagnosed after adverse life events that are not necessarily traumatic. For example, a person showing emotional distress in the aftermath of relationship breakdown, job loss, or illness may warrant a diagnosis of AD; these events would not qualify for a diagnosis of ASD. The person may even have symptoms that resemble ASD—intrusive memories, avoidance, or arousal—but these would not qualify for ASD if the triggering event was not traumatic. The time frames are also different, with ASD not being relevant after 1 month (when PTSD can be diagnosed), and AD requiring the problems to emerge within 3 months of the stressor and usually to resolve within 6 months of its termination. One can also diagnose AD soon after the event occurred. Finally, and possibly most importantly, whereas ASD is an anxiety-focused disorder, AD is very loosely defined and can involve an array of anxiety, mood, or other emotional or conduct problems.

It is not surprising that people can be depressed in the immediate aftermath of trauma exposure. Some level of depression can be expected in most people with ASD, and if it persists for more than 2 weeks, then a formal diagnosis of major depression may also be warranted. Comorbidity can occur, and therefore the clinician need not choose between one diagnosis or the other; however, it is also important that depression is not overdiagnosed as a result of confusing symptoms with ASD. Both conditions will often involve intrusive mental content, but in depression this tends to be more of ruminative dwelling on the traumatic event rather than the anxiety-producing reliving that is normally seen in ASD.

Panic attacks are also very common after trauma and often occur in the context of ASD (Bryant and Panasetis 2001). Some work has shown that these panic attacks are often triggered by trauma reminders and often elicit fears of being unable to cope with the trauma memory (Joscelyne et al. 2012). These reactions can be distinguished from panic disorder by the latter's persistent fear of the consequences of the panic itself, often arising from fear of physical consequences of somatic aberrations that may be experienced.

As indicated by their presence in the DSM criteria, dissociative symptoms commonly occur in ASD. It is possible for a patient to present in the acute phase after trauma without the anxiety symptoms associated with ASD but nonetheless have salient dissociative responses, including fugue states, derealization, or amnesia. If these dissociative reactions are the only presenting problems, these individuals could be diagnosed with depersonalization/derealization disorder or dissociative amnesia. Such presentations are exceptionally rare and should be repeatedly assessed to determine whether more common ASD symptoms are present before making such a diagnosis.

RISK FACTORS FOR ACUTE STRESS DISORDER

Much less work has been done on understanding the risk factors for ASD than for PTSD. Nonetheless, given that the two disorders overlap in so many ways, it is reasonable to assume that many of the same predictors apply to ASD as to PTSD. The following are risk factors for ASD:

- Having a history of prior psychiatric disorder
- Having a history of prior traumatic exposures
- Being female
- Having experienced more severe trauma
- Displaying high levels of neuroticism
- Possessing an avoidant coping style

DSM-5 CRITERIA FOR ACUTE STRESS DISORDER

The definition of ASD changed quite markedly for DSM-5 (Box 5–1) as a result of the work conducted after the introduction of ASD in DSM-IV. One of the most striking shifts was the explicit goal that ASD was no longer intended to predict those individuals who would develop subsequent PTSD. This decision was made because of the evidence that the predictive capacity of the ASD diagnosis was limited. Instead, the emphasis was placed on simply identifying people in the month after trauma exposure who were displaying marked posttraumatic stress and for whom a formal diagnosis may facilitate access to mental health care.

Box 5–1. DSM-5 Diagnostic Criteria for Acute Stress Disorder

308.3 (F43.0)

A. Exposure to actual or threatened death, serious injury, or sexual violation in one (or more) of the following ways:

1. Directly experiencing the traumatic event(s).
2. Witnessing, in person, the event(s) as it occurred to others.
3. Learning that the event(s) occurred to a close family member or close friend. **Note:** In cases of actual or threatened death of a family member or friend, the event(s) must have been violent or accidental.
4. Experiencing repeated or extreme exposure to aversive details of the traumatic event(s) (e.g., first responders collecting human remains, police officers repeatedly exposed to details of child abuse).

   Note: This does not apply to exposure through electronic media, television, movies, or pictures, unless this exposure is work related.

B. Presence of nine (or more) of the following symptoms from any of the five categories of intrusion, negative mood, dissociation, avoidance, and arousal, beginning or worsening after the traumatic event(s) occurred:

Intrusion Symptoms

1. Recurrent, involuntary, and intrusive distressing memories of the traumatic event(s). **Note:** In children, repetitive play may occur in which themes or aspects of the traumatic event(s) are expressed.
2. Recurrent distressing dreams in which the content and/or affect of the dream are related to the event(s). **Note:** In children, there may be frightening dreams without recognizable content.
3. Dissociative reactions (e.g., flashbacks) in which the individual feels or acts as if the traumatic event(s) were recurring. (Such reactions may occur on a continuum, with the most extreme expression being a complete loss of awareness of present surroundings.) **Note:** In children, trauma-specific reenactment may occur in play.
4. Intense or prolonged psychological distress or marked physiological reactions in response to internal or external cues that symbolize or resemble an aspect of the traumatic event(s).

Negative Mood

5. Persistent inability to experience positive emotions (e.g., inability to experience happiness, satisfaction, or loving feelings).

Dissociative Symptoms

6. An altered sense of the reality of one's surroundings or oneself (e.g., seeing oneself from another's perspective, being in a daze, time slowing).
7. Inability to remember an important aspect of the traumatic event(s) (typically due to dissociative amnesia and not to other factors such as head injury, alcohol, or drugs).

Avoidance Symptoms

8. Efforts to avoid distressing memories, thoughts, or feelings about or closely associated with the traumatic event(s).
9. Efforts to avoid external reminders (people, places, conversations, activities, objects, situations) that arouse distressing memories, thoughts, or feelings about or closely associated with the traumatic event(s).

Arousal Symptoms

10. Sleep disturbance (e.g., difficulty falling or staying asleep, restless sleep).
11. Irritable behavior and angry outbursts (with little or no provocation), typically expressed as verbal or physical aggression toward people or objects.
12. Hypervigilance.
13. Problems with concentration.
14. Exaggerated startle response.

C. Duration of the disturbance (symptoms in Criterion B) is 3 days to 1 month after trauma exposure.

Note: Symptoms typically begin immediately after the trauma, but persistence for at least 3 days and up to a month is needed to meet disorder criteria.

D. The disturbance causes clinically significant distress or impairment in social, occupational, or other important areas of functioning.

E. The disturbance is not attributable to the physiological effects of a substance (e.g., medication or alcohol) or another medical condition (e.g., mild traumatic brain injury) and is not better explained by brief psychotic disorder.

Source. Reprinted from the *Diagnostic and Statistical Manual of Mental Disorders,* 5th Edition. Arlington, VA, American Psychiatric Association, 2013. Used with permission. Copyright © 2013 American Psychiatric Association.

One issue considered for DSM-5 was whether ASD should be limited to fear-based posttraumatic stress responses or broadened to include other psychological responses. This consideration was stimulated in part by the broadening of the PTSD definition to include a symptom cluster that described pervasive negative mood states (e.g., anger, shame). Although proponents of the ASD expansion argued it would make the ASD diagnosis more relevant to a larger proportion of trauma survivors, the DSM-5 work group decided not to proceed with this shift in scope because it does not lead to targeted treatment options. As discussed later in the section "Interventions for Treating Acute Stress Disorder," strong evidence supports exposure-based psychotherapy for individuals experiencing ASD, and a broader definition of ASD could make this focused intervention less meaningful for those who present with distress that is not anxiety based. The AD diagnosis was available to capture these other presentations.

There was also a major structural change undertaken in DSM-5 relative to DSM-IV in how the symptoms were configured. This change involved abandoning the requirement that specific symptom clusters be satisfied and instead requiring a minimum number of symptoms—regardless of the permutation of these symptoms. Specifically, the DSM-5 criteria require 9 out of a possible 14 symptoms to be present. This shift was adopted because of evidence that requiring people to satisfy specific clusters may not be appropriate in the acute phase to identify acute stress trauma survivors. In DSM-5 these symptoms need to be evident in the initial month after trauma rather than during the event itself. This was a challenge for the new definition because it required determining a cutoff by which abnormal stress reactions could be distinguished from normal ones. To achieve this, available data sets (comprising more than 3,000 patients) were collated and it was found that 9 symptoms identified approximately 20% of people, and they were characterized by having more distress or impairment relative to those who had fewer than 9 symptoms (Bryant et al. 2011).

Numerous changes also were made in DSM-5 to ensure that ASD criteria were as close as possible to changes made to the PTSD criteria. The DSM-IV

Criterion A2 (requiring "fear, helplessness, or horror") was removed from the PTSD and ASD criteria because of evidence that it does not enhance identification of individuals with PTSD (Brewin et al. 2000), and it even excludes those who would otherwise satisfy PTSD criteria. Many critics have argued that this criterion is not appropriate for some military personnel, who may not experience fear at the time of trauma exposure because they are focused on their duties, or for patients who sustain a mild traumatic brain injury and suffer transient loss of consciousness. Also, some dissociative symptoms were deleted (reduced awareness of one's surroundings) or combined (derealization and depersonalization) because of evidence that they either are limited to experiences during the trauma or typically coexist and therefore do not enhance diagnostic accuracy.

The patient in the following dialogue presented to the clinic where I work following a vicious assault in which bandits entered the home where he lived alone. They held him hostage, and threatened his life. This person was referred for treatment 2 weeks after the incident. I present here an excerpt from the initial assessment, which includes the patient's account of his experience and presenting problems.

> **Patient:** Since it happened 2 weeks ago, I cannot get it out of my mind. I keep replaying it over and over in my head. I try to stop it, but these images are always there.
>
> **Therapist:** What images?
>
> **Patient:** I see blood. I can't talk about it, but I see all this blood everywhere. I am trying to block it out, but it is just images of red. It scares the hell out of me. And everything triggers it off. I can't even cook meat anymore because there is red juice in it—it looks just like the blood.
>
> **Therapist:** What else about the experience do you find yourself thinking about?
>
> **Patient:** Nothing. I don't allow myself. It is weird, but the main memory I have is of the blood. Just pools of my blood. Exactly what happened, I don't know. It is all a blur. In the hospital they asked me if I was knocked out because there was so much detail I could not remember, but I wasn't. I just don't remember so much. But I also don't think I want to.
>
> **Therapist:** You mentioned you try to block these memories out? What do you do to block these out?
>
> **Patient:** Whatever it takes. I am not eating meat. I can't watch TV or read anything about crime or war. It brings it all back. And I never feel safe. I have put new locks on all my doors, but it is not enough. I am planning to sell my place and move. I need to get out of the city. I cannot be safe here. Maybe somewhere in the country would be better. And I haven't slept since it happened. My doctor gave me sleeping pills, but then the nightmares start. I see the whole thing again and I wake screaming. So it is better to stay up most of the night than have those dreams.
>
> **Therapist:** What else has been troubling you?
>
> **Patient:** Don't know if this is normal, but I am so jumpy. Anything sets me off. If there is noise anywhere, I jump. The other day the phone rang at home and I nearly hit the roof. I get really scared, but I also get really angry.

These guys had no right doing those things to me, but I am getting really aggressive at everyone now. The other day this woman put me on hold on the phone and I tore shreds off her. This is not like me.

Therapist: How has it affected your day-to-day life at the moment?

Patient: Well, I am not the same person. I try not to go out because I am scared. When I do, I make sure I see everyone around me. The other day I went into a coffee shop to meet my brother, and I insisted on sitting with my back to the wall so I could see everyone. I can't bear to think someone is coming behind me. To be honest, I spend most of my time at my brother's place because I cannot be at home. Too many things there remind me of what happened. Every time I try to go home and I put my key in the lock, I am sure these guys are behind the door. So often I have gone home but then turned away and gone back to my brother's.

The patient in this account displays many of the classic symptoms of ASD. He is frequently reexperiencing the event, is highly avoidant of reminders of the trauma, and is clearly agitated and hypervigilant. His pattern of engaging in excessive safety behaviors is very typical of ASD patients and reflects their need to regain a sense of control. This patient's description of patchy memories reflects a degree of dissociative amnesia. It is difficult to know whether he did or did not initially encode this information, but the global nature of his poor recall suggests that he is avoiding remembering what transpired.

EPIDEMIOLOGY OF ACUTE STRESS DISORDER

Population estimates of ASD are difficult to determine because there is a limited time in which the diagnosis can be made. Moreover, because of the time pressure placed on population-level psychiatric surveys, ASD is typically not included in the studies using those surveys. More information is available about the incidence of ASD following different types of traumatic events. In the systematic review of longitudinal studies of ASD (Bryant 2011), the rates of ASD were found to vary from 7% to 59%, with an average of 19%. Considering that one function of ASD is to identify people in the acute phase who suffer severe posttraumatic stress, these rates appear to satisfy this goal. Nine studies reported "subsyndromal" ASD (which was typically defined as satisfying three of the four DSM-IV symptom clusters). When this definition is used, the rates unsurprisingly increase to a range of 10%–66% and an average of 26%. In terms of specific trauma types, ASD has been reported following motor vehicle accidents (13%–21%), mild traumatic brain injury (14%), assault (16%–19%), burns (10%), industrial accidents (6%), and witnessing of a mass shooting (33%).

INTERVENTIONS FOR TREATING ACUTE STRESS DISORDER

Psychotherapy Approaches

Without doubt, the treatment for ASD with the most empirical support is trauma-focused cognitive-behavioral therapy (CBT). It is the recommended treatment across a number of treatment guidelines (Foa et al. 2009). This modality usually commences with psychoeducation about the trauma responses and then focuses on anxiety management, exposure, and cognitive restructuring. Psychoeducation is used to instruct the patient about common posttraumatic stress symptoms and the way in which the core symptoms are treated in therapy. Anxiety management aims to reduce anxiety through a range of techniques, including breathing retraining, relaxation skills, and self-talk. Exposure therapy is arguably the key ingredient in treatment and optimally involves both imaginal and in vivo exposure. In imaginal exposure, the patient is asked to vividly recall his or her traumatic experience for protracted periods, usually for at least 30 minutes. The patient provides a narrative of the traumatic experience, including descriptions of sensory cues and affective responses. This exercise is typically commenced during therapy sessions and continued as homework between sessions. In vivo exposure involves graded exposure to feared stimuli; the patient is initially asked to remain in proximity to minimally fearful reminders of the trauma, and then this exercise is repeated with increasingly fearful situations until the person feels comfortable with most reminders of the experience. In cognitive restructuring, the therapist works with the patient to evaluate how realistic negative automatic thoughts are and to develop cognitive strategies to reappraise them.

Most exposure-based approaches have developed from fear conditioning, the central mechanism underpinning the development and resolution of posttraumatic stress. In this model, cues present during a traumatic event are paired with strong fear reactions, which in turn lead to conditioned fear responses, which then activate fear networks when the individual is exposed to these reminders (Foa et al. 1989). When reminders of the trauma occur, people respond with fear reactions and reexperiencing symptoms. Fear conditioning models propose that successful recovery from trauma involves *extinction learning*, in which repeated exposure to trauma reminders or memories results in new learning that these reminders no longer signal threat. In the laboratory, for example, a rat might be repeatedly exposed to a light that was previously conditioned with an electric shock, and as the rat learns that the light no longer signals threat, it no longer has a fear reaction to it. A rape victim with ASD may be repeatedly exposed to memories of the assault, but as the woman learns that these memories no longer harm her, she no longer has the anxiety response. Similarly, in the course of in vivo exposure, the rape victim may begin talking to men again and repeatedly learn that they are not attacking her, thereby achieving extinction learning and remission of symptoms.

More cognitively oriented models emphasize that appraisals of the traumatic event and associated symptoms are the key etiological and maintaining factors, and, accordingly, these approaches tend to emphasize cognitive elements of CBT (Ehlers and Clark 2000). In support of this view is evidence that people with ASD exaggerate both the probability of future negative events occurring and the adverse effects of these events (Warda and Bryant 1998). Moreover, patients with ASD display cognitive biases for a range of events beyond those directly related to the traumatic experience, including external harm, somatic sensations, and social concerns (Smith and Bryant 2000). Additionally, excessively negative appraisals made in the initial month after trauma predict subsequent PTSD (Dunmore et al. 2001).

Psychotherapy for ASD: Review of the Evidence

Traditional approaches of trauma-focused CBT for PTSD have been adapted over the past 20 years to address ASD. Specifically, these approaches have usually been abridged so that therapy is provided in five to six sessions, and they usually commence several weeks after trauma exposure. In the first study of this approach to treat ASD, patients who had survived motor vehicle accidents or assault were randomly assigned to either CBT or nondirective supportive counseling (Bryant et al. 1998). Both interventions consisted of five 1.5-hour weekly individual therapy sessions. The CBT included education about posttraumatic reactions, relaxation training, cognitive restructuring, and both imaginal and in vivo exposure to the traumatic event. The supportive counseling condition included trauma education and more general problem-solving skills training. At 6-month follow-up, fewer participants had PTSD in the CBT group (20%) than in the supportive counseling control group (67%). This superiority of CBT over more nondirective counseling has been reported in numerous trials since that study, with the treatment gains of those who received CBT being maintained 4 years after treatment. Reflecting the potential effectiveness of CBT for ASD is the finding of a meta-analysis that early provision of CBT was superior to comparative interventions (Roberts et al. 2009).

A couple of early-intervention studies are worth noting because they point to important issues that need to be considered in the treatment of ASD. In a large study, 90 trauma survivors were assigned to receive either five weekly sessions of imaginal and in vivo exposure, cognitive restructuring, or assessment only (Bryant et al. 2008). Findings indicated that individuals receiving exposure therapy had lower levels of PTSD, depression, and anxiety at posttreatment and follow-up than did subjects in the other conditions. This study suggests that it is important to ensure that patients engage in emotional processing of the trauma memory to achieve optimal treatment gains. In a very large study conducted in Israel, Shalev et al. (2012) randomly assigned 242 patients admitted to an emergency department who met criteria for either full or subsyndromal ASD to one of the following: prolonged exposure, cognitive restructuring, waitlist, a selective serotonin reuptake inhibitor (SSRI), or placebo. (Those in the waitlist group were randomly assigned to exposure or cognitive restructuring after 12 weeks.) Nine months after treatment, PTSD rates were comparable across exposure (21%) and cognitive restructuring (22%) conditions. Very interestingly, there were no long-term differences between participants who received the early or later provision of CBT. This finding suggests that the need to treat people in the very early phase is not as crucial as people often think, because patients tended to achieve comparable levels of PTSD symptomatology whether they received early or later intervention.

The following is an example of imaginal exposure with a patient (using the same example of the patient provided earlier).

Therapist: Now, as I mentioned earlier, we are going to tackle the memory of what happened that night. I know others have asked you about it before, like the police, but I want us to relive it differently. I don't want you to give me a factual account of what happened. Instead, I want you to really relive the experience. I want you to think and imagine closely what happened, what you saw and heard, even what you smelled or touched. Most importantly, I want you to tell me what you were feeling. It helps if you can talk in the first person using words like *I* and *me* and keep it present rather than past. Some people find this easier to do with their eyes closed. Also, I want to know how you are feeling but I don't want to interrupt you. So I am going to ask you to describe to me now and then how you are feeling using a scale, on which 1 means that you do not feel at all distressed and 100 means that you feel extremely distressed. So when I ask you how you are feeling, you can just tell me a number that best describes how you are feeling. OK, you can start now.

Patient: I was watching TV when suddenly the door burst open with an incredible crash and these three men with hoods on their heads came in. They were carrying clubs and knives. One of them picked me up and threw me against the wall. He later cut me....

Therapist: Wait a minute. You are telling me as if it is in the past. I know this is unusual, but can you describe it to me as if it is happening here and now?

Patient: Right. I forgot. So the next thing I know is that I am being thrown against a wall. I feel my head thumping against a light fitting, and it immediately feels wet. Straight away I know I am bleeding. My mind is racing. I don't know why these guys are here. I don't have much money. I don't have drugs. I try telling them to take whatever they want. But they just laugh at me. They sit down in my chairs as if they own the place as I am curled up on the floor. Then one of them comes over to me and kicks me in the head. His boot hits me right in the mouth. I can feel a tooth give way and my mouth fills up with blood. He is bending over and puts his head right next to my ear. He then whispers to me, "We don't want your money. We just want to have some fun with you." This is terrible. I want to stop.

Therapist: I understand. This is never easy. But you are doing yourself good by doing this. We are getting a handle on the memory. Can you tell me how you are feeling right now on that scale of 1–100?

Patient: Shocking. I am at 100.

Therapist: All right. The main thing is that you are staying with it. And you can see we are both here and surviving this. I would like you to continue and tell me what is happening next. You really are doing this very well.

Patient: Well, the next thing is what really gets to me. One of the guys pulls out a knife and cuts my pants off. He is not taking any care. He is just slashing away at the legs of my pants. I can feel him cutting my legs repeatedly. I am praying he is not hitting veins because I know I am going to die. They are laughing at the pool of blood building up around me. I can feel myself lying in my own blood. It is so red. So deep red. I can't stand this. Why are they doing this to me? Why? And then another guy takes the knife off the guy and holds it at my penis. They are daring him to cut it off. I shut my eyes—waiting for it to happen. I need to stop. I can't continue.

Therapist: All right. You are doing really well. What is your rating on that scale now?

Patient: Still 100.

Therapist: I want us to continue. But I want you to move onto the next bit of what happened that you are OK talking about today. You choose.

Patient: All right. It is about half an hour later. They have me sitting up on a chair. Naked. I am staring at them as they paint my walls with my own blood. They are soaking it up from the floor and wiping it all over the place. This is making me sick. I am feeling dizzy. I am thinking I am losing so much blood I cannot stay awake. Everything is getting very dreamy. And then I pass out, I guess. Sometime later I wake up. No idea how long it is, but there are two paramedics kneeling over me. They are working hard. They look worried but they keep telling me I am safe now. That's it.

Therapist: And how do you feel now on the scale?

Patient: I guess about 90. It has come down a bit. I never thought it would.

Therapist: OK. Now I want you to know that you did really well on that. But I really want you to leave here today making as many gains as you can. So we are going to do this one more time. You can focus on the same things as you did just then, or you may find yourself recalling more details. We will see.

The session would normally then repeat the exposure, with the goal that the patient stays close to the memory for at least 30 minutes. The patient would then be asked to commence doing the exposure for homework. The intent is that the patient's subsequent exposure sessions eventually cover all aspects of the experience, even those that were initially avoided.

Pharmacological Approaches

Very few controlled pharmacological trials have been reported in the ASD literature, although there have been a number of open trials that lack full methodological
rigor. The most compelling study to date is the Israeli study mentioned in the previous section. In that study of early intervention, the 242 patients were randomly assigned to prolonged exposure, cognitive restructuring, waitlist, the SSRI
escitalopram, or placebo (Shalev et al. 2012). At 9-month follow-up, PTSD rates in
both exposure (21%) and restructuring (22%) conditions were lower than rates in
the SSRI (42%) and placebo (47%) conditions. The lesson from this trial is that escitalopram does not perform markedly better than placebo in treating PTSD. Moreover, given that this SSRI is a commonly recommended antidepressant for treatment
of PTSD, it may not have meaningful benefits for patients with ASD either.

FUTURE OF ACUTE STRESS DISORDER

Although the history of ASD has been brief and controversial, scientifically rich and
clinically useful research and applied activity have been done. The innovations that
have occurred since ASD was introduced in 1994 will no doubt continue as researchers continue to seek novel pharmacological and psychological means to limit
psychopathological responses to trauma. It is probable that some of the most sophisticated developments will come as a result of new advancements in statistical
approaches that can model the trajectories of posttraumatic adjustment over the
immediate and longer-term phases, and these statistical approaches will probably
highlight the complexity and heterogeneity of acute and chronic response rather
than its simplicity. More sophisticated statistical studies of posttraumatic stress response will probably bring new challenges because practitioners in the field of posttraumatic stress will need to understand the complex array of responses, develop
appropriate ways to predict which patients will follow different pathways, and tailor
treatments to meet the divergent needs of patients. (ICD-11 does not plan to include ASD in its central taxonomy. See Chapter 11, "ICD-10, ICD-11, and DSM-5.")

Key Points

- Acute stress disorder (ASD) was introduced in DSM-IV to describe severe acute stress reactions after trauma and also to
  identify people in the acute phase who are likely to develop
  subsequent posttraumatic stress disorder (PTSD).

- ASD, as defined in DSM-IV, required display of each of the dissociative, reexperiencing, avoidance, and arousal clusters of
  symptoms.

- Longitudinal studies indicate that the ASD diagnosis does not adequately identify most people who develop PTSD.

- In DSM-5, ASD was reconceptualized so that its goal was to identify people with severe acute stress reactions but not to identify people who are at high risk for developing PTSD.

- In DSM-5, ASD diagnosis requires that a minimum of 9 of the potential 14 symptoms are present at least 3 days after trauma.

- There is convincing evidence that treating ASD with brief trauma-focused cognitive-behavioral therapy limits subsequent PTSD in most people.

SUGGESTED READINGS

Bryant RA: Acute stress disorder as a predictor of posttraumatic stress disorder: a systematic review. J Clin Psychiatry 72(2):233–239, 2011 21208593

Bryant RA, Friedman MJ, Spiegel D, et al: A review of acute stress disorder in DSM-5. Depress Anxiety 28(9):802–817, 2011 21910186

Cardeña E, Carlson E: Acute stress disorder revisited. Annu Rev Clin Psychol 7:245–267. 2011 21275643

Harvey AG, Bryant RA: Acute stress disorder: a synthesis and critique. Psychol Bull 128(6):886–902, 2002 12405136

REFERENCES

American Psychiatric Association: Diagnostic and Statistical Manual of Mental Disorders, 4th Edition. Washington, DC, American Psychiatric Association, 1994

American Psychiatric Association: Diagnostic and Statistical Manual of Mental Disorders, 5th Edition. Arlington, VA, American Psychiatric Association 2013

Brewin CR, Andrews B, Rose S: Fear, helplessness, and horror in posttraumatic stress disorder: investigating DSM-IV criterion A2 in victims of violent crime. J Trauma Stress 13(3):499–509, 2000 10948489

Briere J, Scott C, Weathers F: Peritraumatic and persistent dissociation in the presumed etiology of PTSD. Am J Psychiatry 162(12):2295–2301, 2005 16330593

Bryant RA: Early predictors of posttraumatic stress disorder. Biol Psychiatry 53(9):789–795, 2003 12725971

Bryant RA: Acute stress disorder as a predictor of posttraumatic stress disorder: a systematic review. J Clin Psychiatry 72(2):233–239, 2011 21208593

Bryant RA, Harvey AG: Acute stress disorder: a critical review of diagnostic issues. Clin Psychol Rev 17(7):757–773, 1997 9397336

Bryant RA, Harvey AG: New DSM-IV diagnosis of acute stress disorder. Am J Psychiatry 157(11):1889–1891, 2000 11058505

Bryant RA, Panasetis P: Panic symptoms during trauma and acute stress disorder. Behav Res Ther 39(8):961–966, 2001 11480836

Bryant RA, Harvey AG, Dang ST, et al: Treatment of acute stress disorder: a comparison of cognitive-behavioral therapy and supportive counseling. J Consult Clin Psychol 66(5):862–866, 1998 9803707

Bryant RA, Mastrodomenico J, Felmingham KL, et al: Treatment of acute stress disorder: a randomized controlled trial. Arch Gen Psychiatry 65(6):659–667, 2008 18519824

Bryant RA, Friedman MJ, Spiegel D, et al: A review of acute stress disorder in DSM-5. Depress Anxiety 28(9):802–817, 2011 21910186

Bryant RA, O'Donnell ML, Creamer M, et al: A multisite analysis of the fluctuating course of posttraumatic stress disorder. JAMA Psychiatry 70(8):839–846, 2013 23784521

Dunmore E, Clark DM, Ehlers A: A prospective investigation of the role of cognitive factors in persistent posttraumatic stress disorder (PTSD) after physical or sexual assault. Behav Res Ther 39(9):1063–1084, 2001 11520012

Ehlers A, Clark DM: A cognitive model of posttraumatic stress disorder. Behav Res Ther 38(4):319–345, 2000 10761279

Ehlers A, Mayou RA, Bryant B: Psychological predictors of chronic posttraumatic stress disorder after motor vehicle accidents. J Abnorm Psychol 107(3):508–519, 1998 9715585

Foa EB, Steketee G, Rothbaum BO: Behavioral/cognitive conceptualizations of post-traumatic stress disorder. Behav Ther 20:155–176, 1989

Foa EB, Keane TM, Friedman MJ, et al: Effective Treatments for PTSD: Practice Guide-lines From the International Society of Traumatic Stress Studies, 2nd Edition. New York, Guilford, 2009

Joscelyne A, McLean S, Drobny J, et al: Fear of memories: the nature of panic in post-traumatic stress disorder. Eur J Psychotraumatol 3, DOI: 10.3402/ejpt.v3i0.19084, 2012 [Epub] 23130094

Koopman C, Classen C, Cardeña E, et al: When disaster strikes, acute stress disorder may follow. J Trauma Stress 8(1):29–46, 1995 7712057

Marshall RD, Spitzer R, Liebowitz MR: Review and critique of the new DSM-IV diagno-sis of acute stress disorder. Am J Psychiatry 156(11):1677–1685, 1999 10553729

Murray J, Ehlers A, Mayou RA: Dissociation and post-traumatic stress disorder: two prospective studies of road traffic accident survivors. Br J Psychiatry 180:363–368, 2002 11925361

Roberts NP, Kitchiner NJ, Kenardy J, et al: Systematic review and meta-analysis of mul-tiple-session early interventions following traumatic events. Am J Psychiatry 166(3):293–301, 2009 19188285

Shalev AY, Ankri Y, Israeli-Shalev Y, et al: Prevention of posttraumatic stress disorder by early treatment: results from the Jerusalem Trauma Outreach and Prevention study. Arch Gen Psychiatry 69(2):166–176, 2012 21969418

Simeon D, Guralnik O: New DSM-IV diagnosis of acute stress disorder. Am J Psychiatry 157(11):1888–1889, author reply 1890–1891, 2000 11058503

Smith K, Bryant RA: The generality of cognitive bias in acute stress disorder. Behav Res Ther 38(7):709–715, 2000 10875192

Spiegel D, Koopman C, Classen C: Acute stress disorder and dissociation. Aust Clin Ex-periment Hypn 22:11–23, 1994

Spiegel D, Classen C, Cardeña E: New DSM-IV diagnosis of acute stress disorder. Am J Psychiatry 157(11):1890–1891, 2000 11058507

Warda G, Bryant RA: Cognitive bias in acute stress disorder. Behav Res Ther 36(12):1177–1183, 1998 9745802

CHAPTER 6

Posttraumatic Stress Disorder

EPIDEMIOLOGY, DIAGNOSIS, AND TREATMENT

AMY LEHRNER, PH.D.
LAURA C. PRATCHETT, PSY.D.
RACHEL YEHUDA, PH.D.

POSTTRAUMATIC STRESS disorder (PTSD) was first codified as a mental disorder in 1980 in DSM-III (American Psychiatric Association 1980). However, acute and chronic symptoms following traumatic experiences have been observed since the time of Herodotus (the so-called father of history in the fifth century B.C.), particularly among war veterans. Pronounced and disabling consequences of war have been termed "soldier's heart," traumatic neurosis, shell shock, and combat neurosis (Yehuda and McFarlane 1995). Although these symptoms were expected to resolve on their own following a period of rest and recuperation, it became increasingly clear that some trauma survivors continued to suffer over long periods of time. With DSM-III, PTSD was reframed as a normative response to a trauma outside the realm of normal experience: "The stressor producing this syndrome would evoke significant symptoms of distress in most people, and is generally outside the range of such common experiences as simple bereavement, chronic illness, business losses, or marital conflict" (American Psychiatric Association 1980, p. 236).

Epidemiological research has now clarified that although a precipitating trauma may indeed provoke distressing initial symptoms, most people do in fact show resilience and recover naturally without intervention (see Chapter 9, "Therapeutic Adaptations of Resilience"). Of those exposed to a traumatic experience, 15%–25% develop significant symptoms that meet diagnostic criteria for PTSD (Riggs et al. 1995; Rothbaum et al. 1992). The likelihood of developing PTSD after trauma exposure varies by population, individual risk factors, and type of trauma. For example, there are higher prevalence rates (approximately one-third to one-half) among individuals exposed to rape, combat, and genocide. Overall, approximately 6.8% of adults—3.6% of men and 9.7% of women—in the United States are estimated to experience PTSD in their lifetimes (Kessler et al. 2005; National Comorbidity Survey 2005). It is unknown why women have higher rates of PTSD following trauma than men; theories include biological (e.g., hormonal), psychological, and sociological (e.g., women are more likely to experience interpersonal violence and sexual assault that occur in close relationships and that involve a betrayal of trust) reasons (Pratchett et al. 2010). Longitudinal research has identified multiple posttrauma trajectories, which generally include resilience as the most common trajectory, recovery, chronic symptoms, and delayed onset of symptoms. Trajectory models vary on the basis of the population, with evidence that pretrauma, peritrauma, and posttrauma risk or protective factors influence trajectory membership. For example, individuals trained to respond in emergency or combat situations (e.g., police, soldiers) may exhibit more resilience following trauma exposure (Pietrzak et al. 2014). Symptoms may wax and wane and may be influenced by external influences (e.g., trauma anniversaries, other life stressors, or protective factors such as social support) as well as by behavioral factors such as substance use.

CLASSIFICATION

Prior to DSM-5 (American Psychiatric Association 2013), PTSD was categorized as an anxiety disorder on the basis of similar symptom presentations across anxiety disorders. For example, PTSD symptoms include anxious arousal that takes the form of hypervigilance and increased startle reaction. Individuals with PTSD frequently experience panic symptoms or full-blown attacks when triggered by trauma reminders and agoraphobic avoidance behavior to minimize exposure to trauma reminders. Recurrent intrusive thoughts or images that are unwanted and unpleasant can present similarly to obsessional thoughts in obsessive-compulsive disorder. However, PTSD symptoms also overlap with depression criteria, including anhedonia, insomnia, and difficulty concentrating, as reflected by the high comorbidity of PTSD and major depressive disorder. Symptoms of clinical distress following trauma may include anxiety and fear, depressive symptoms, angry and aggressive behaviors, or dissociative symptoms. In recognition of these multiple clinical phenotypes and the etiological prerequisite of trauma exposure, DSM-5 has included PTSD under a new classification: trauma- and stressor-related disorders.

DIAGNOSTIC CRITERIA

Fundamental to epidemiological estimates and psychiatric diagnosis is the definition of a precipitating traumatic event. Stress and trauma disorders are unique in their requirement of an environmental stressor for diagnosis. Among the alterations to the PTSD criteria in DSM-5 is a more stringent criterion for what is considered a qualifying index trauma (Criterion A)—that is, the nature of the experience that is considered sufficiently traumatic to result in the specific pathological responses conceptualized as PTSD. Accordingly, events experienced as intensely distressing or stressful but lacking the shocking nature of a trauma (e.g., the nonviolent or sudden death of a loved one) can no longer be considered Criterion A events. For a PTSD diagnosis, DSM-5 requires "exposure to actual or threatened death, serious injury, or sexual violence" (p. 271). This exposure may take the form of direct personal exposure, in-person witnessing, indirect exposure (i.e., learning that a close relative or friend was exposed to trauma, which, if involving death or threat of death, must have been "violent or accidental"), or "repeated or extreme indirect exposure to aversive details of the traumatic event(s)" (e.g., as a professional). DSM-5 explicitly excludes nonprofessional exposure through the media or other images. Although other experiences may feel "traumatic" and have real emotional and psychological consequences (e.g., divorce, infidelity, death of a loved one due to illness), they do not qualify as a Criterion A trauma for PTSD. Diagnoses such as adjustment disorder, major depressive disorder, or other specified trauma- and stressor-related disorder should be considered for clinically significant symptoms following such experiences.

Another change is the removal of the DSM-IV Criterion A2, which specified that a Criterion A trauma must elicit feelings of "intense fear, helplessness, or horror" (American Psychiatric Association 1994, p. 428). This criterion reflected the assumption that the intensity of the emotional response is fundamental to the development of the disorder and is an indicator of the severity of the trauma. Research has shown that this criterion did not improve diagnostic accuracy, was not strongly predictive of PTSD, and is vulnerable to recall bias. For example, some people experience numbing or dissociation during a trauma, whereas soldiers are trained to respond on the basis of prior training and to distance themselves from any emotional reactions. There is some evidence that removing the A2 criterion may lead to an increase in prevalence rates, because some studies have found that more than 20% of individuals who met all other diagnostic criteria for PTSD failed to receive a diagnosis because they did not meet Criterion A2 (Friedman et al. 2011).

There are four PTSD symptom clusters in DSM-5, revised from three in DSM-IV. Intrusive symptoms (Criterion B) may include 1) repeated, unwanted, intrusive memories (which may present as repetitive play in children); 2) distressing dreams; 3) dissociative reactions (e.g., flashbacks), which may involve reenactments in children; 4) intense distress at reminders; and 5) strong physiological reactions to reminders. One intrusive symptom is required for diagnosis.

Avoidance and numbing symptoms, previously conceptualized as a single cluster, have been split in DSM-5. Avoidance symptoms (Criterion C) are persistent efforts to avoid 1) thoughts or feelings about the trauma (internal reminders) or 2) external trauma-related stimuli (e.g., people, places, situations, activities, objects). One avoidance symptom is required for diagnosis.

Depressive symptoms of numbing and anhedonia are now incorporated in negative alterations in cognitions and mood (Criterion D), which reflect distressing or maladaptive thought patterns and mood that begin or worsen following the trauma. They may include 1) dissociative amnesia for key aspects of the trauma; 2) persistent negative beliefs about oneself, others, or the world (e.g., that the world is completely dangerous); 3) distorted blame toward self or others for the trauma or the consequences; 4) persistent negative emotions related to the trauma (e.g., fear, anger, guilt, shame); 5) significantly diminished interest in important activities; 6) alienation from others; and 7) constricted affect (inability to experience positive emotions). Two Criterion D symptoms are required for diagnosis.

Alterations in arousal and reactivity (Criterion E) begin or worsen following the trauma, and these may include 1) irritability or aggressive behavior, 2) self-destructive or reckless behavior, 3) hypervigilance, 4) exaggerated startle response, 5) concentration difficulty, or 6) sleep disturbance. Two Criterion D symptoms are required for diagnosis.

Criteria B–E symptoms must persist for more than 1 month and cause significant distress or functional impairment.

Two PTSD specifiers have been added in DSM-5: 1) with dissociative symptoms and 2) with delayed expression. If a patient does not meet full diagnostic criteria until 6 months or longer posttrauma, the delayed expression specifier is appropriate, even if some symptoms have immediate onset. The dissociative specifier applies to individuals who meet the previously listed criteria for diagnosis and additionally have high levels of depersonalization (i.e., feeling that one is an outside observer or detached from one's body; "this is not me") or derealization (i.e., a feeling that things are not real or are distorted; "this is not really happening"). Dissociation represents an extreme state of altered consciousness to defend the self against an intolerable or inescapable experience, allowing an individual to survive and continue to function in the face of an overwhelming trauma such as childhood abuse or torture. Approximately 15%–30% of individuals with PTSD report dissociative symptoms (Wolf et al. 2012). Risk factors for the dissociative specifier include male gender, repeated and early traumatic experiences, and comorbid psychiatric conditions (Stein et al. 2013). These patients have higher rates of suicidality and report more functional impairment (Stein et al. 2013). The inclusion of the dissociative subtype is supported by neurobiological findings that individuals with PTSD who dissociate show opposite patterns of activation in the medial prefrontal cortex and rostral anterior cingulate cortex (increased rather than decreased) compared with those who do not dissociate (Lanius et al. 2012). Dissociation in response to trauma and trauma reminders has been conceptualized as a core symptom of a theorized complex PTSD construct that, although not codified in DSM, has been proposed as a disorder that may result from chronic, interpersonal trauma exposure, particularly starting early in development, such as childhood sexual trauma (Herman 1992). There is some evidence that individuals with dissociative symptoms may respond differentially to trauma-focused therapies and may benefit more from treatments emphasizing cognitive processing (e.g., cognitive processing therapy) and emotion regulation skills (Cloitre et al. 2012; Resick et al. 2012).

RISK FACTORS

PTSD results from a complex interplay of genetic, developmental, endocrine, neurobiological, cognitive, and environmental factors. Risk factors for the development of PTSD following trauma exposure include pretraumatic, peritraumatic, and posttraumatic factors (Brewin et al. 2000; Ozer et al. 2003). Preexisting risk factors include a history (or family history) of psychiatric treatment, emotional problems, or illness, particularly prior PTSD or other anxiety or affective disorders; prior trauma exposure or childhood abuse or adversity; younger age; female gender; low socioeconomic status; and low intelligence or educational attainment. Peritraumatic risk factors include the severity, duration, and chronicity of the trauma and extreme distress or dissociation during the trauma. Posttraumatic risk factors include lack of social support, ongoing stress or continued or new adverse life events, comorbid physical conditions (e.g., traumatic brain injury, pain), and poor coping strategies (e.g., substance abuse, poor sleep hygiene). Biological dysregulation (e.g., increased glucocorticoid sensitivity, low cortisol signaling, elevated heart rate, elevated catecholamines) prior to or during the trauma also confers risk for development of PTSD.

BIOLOGY

Initial hypotheses about PTSD pathophysiology were based on the assumption that PTSD was a prolonged stress response and that biological systems associated with threat and stress, such as the hypothalamic-pituitary-adrenal (HPA) axis, would show heightened activity. However, research now suggests that PTSD represents a failure of the natural stress response cycle, such that lower levels of cortisol and increased glucocorticoid sensitivity suppress the HPA axis, with resulting increased and prolonged sympathetic system activation (Yehuda 2009). HPA axis alterations that occur in PTSD—including low cortisol; increased glucocorticoid sensitivity; higher numbers of glucocorticoid receptors; and higher levels of norepinephrine, corticotropin-releasing hormone (CRH), and proinflammatory cytokines—are all suggestive of a dysregulated glucocorticoid signaling pathway, which may leave individuals more vulnerable to hyperresponsiveness to threat or provocation (Daskalakis et al. 2013; van Zuiden et al. 2013). Other biological abnormalities in PTSD include higher baseline heart rate, blood pressure, and startle responses.

Brain alterations in PTSD have also been observed. The amygdala is important for the acquisition, modulation, and expression of fear memories, and neuroimaging studies have consistently found increased amygdala activity and size and hyperresponsiveness to trauma-related stimuli (Zoladz and Diamond 2013). The prefrontal cortex is responsible for higher-order cognitive functions, including executive function, attention, decision making, and planning. Imaging studies have consistently documented reduced prefrontal cortex size and function in PTSD (Zoladz and Diamond 2013). Lower hippocampal volume has also been reported in PTSD (Pitman et al. 2012). Taken together, functional neuroimaging studies suggest a hyperactive limbic system driven by reduced activity in the anterior cingulate cortex, which may lead to an overreactive amygdala that amplifies fear signaling (Shin and Liberzon 2010).

An enhanced or prolonged response to threat may be adaptive in some environments. However, the failure to contain sympathetic activation precludes a return to homeostasis and increases the risk for other health problems associated with chronic allostatic load and glucocorticoid function, including diabetes and obesity and autoimmune, cardiovascular, and gastrointestinal diseases (Boscarino 2004; Qureshi et al. 2009).

Recent research has sought to identify relevant "upstream" molecular and genetic factors and pathways that may influence risk and disease processes that have been associated with PTSD, such as increased glucocorticoid sensitivity (Neylan et al. 2014). Such factors include genetic polymorphisms and epigenetic modifications affecting gene expression, and genes such as the glucocorticoid receptor gene NR3C1 (nuclear receptor subfamily 3, group C, member 1), the CRH type 1 receptor gene CRHR1, and the FK506 binding protein 5 gene FKBP5 have been associated with PTSD. As such pathways and networks are identified, potentially mutable treatment targets are being pursued. Future pharmacological interventions may attempt to boost resilience prior to trauma exposure (primary prevention) or immediately following exposure (secondary prevention), and new treatments for the disorder are being investigated. Early investigations of propranolol did not find evidence of prophylaxis, but preliminary studies have shown that administration of cortisol in the acute aftermath of trauma may have preventive effects (Amos et al. 2014).

ASSESSMENT AND DIAGNOSIS

Patients often do not spontaneously report trauma history or link current symptoms with trauma exposure. Patients may present with symptoms, such as mood swings, anxiety, irritability, insomnia, or relationship problems, that they do not associate with trauma exposure, and the identification of a traumatic stressor may be complicated by the patient's efforts to avoid talking or thinking about the trauma. However, failure to identify PTSD can lead to ineffective treatment, poor rapport, and treatment noncompliance and dropout. Providers should directly assess new patients for trauma exposure, including type, frequency, and severity of the experience(s).

When a patient's trauma history is identified, providers should screen for PTSD symptoms. There are a number of well-validated self-report or clinician-administered screening measures that can be used (for information and links to screening tools, see the National Center for PTSD Web site, listed in "Suggested Readings and Web Sites" at the end of this chapter). Only one of these tools, however, has been revised to date for DSM-5: the PTSD Checklist for DSM-5 (PCL-5; Weathers et al. 2013). On the PCL-5, the current suggested cutoff score for a positive screen is 38 (pending possible revision following further validation studies). Patients who have a positive screen for PTSD should be more fully assessed. Relevant information includes length of time since trauma exposure; nature, frequency, and intensity of symptoms; and degree of social and functional impairment.

When assessing for PTSD symptoms, the clinician should consider that the majority of individuals who experience trauma do not develop PTSD. Other mental health consequences, including depression, anxiety, substance use disorders, and personality disorders, are all common, and diagnosis and assessment should carefully delineate between PTSD and other trauma-related sequelae. Because these disorders are also commonly comorbid with PTSD, this process can be challenging at times. Cultural and religious background may also influence symptom presentation and should be considered with all patients and in particular with immigrant, refugee, or minority populations.

The clinician needs to link the individual's experience of any reported symptoms to the actual experience of trauma, but this can be challenging at times and requires a nonleading approach that does not presume PTSD. Symptoms of avoidance, emotional and cognitive changes, and hyperarousal may present in individuals with trauma histories without being consequences of the trauma exposure, so follow-up questions to identify the link are necessary. A number of challenges also can exist in the exploration of reexperiencing symptoms. One common challenge, which the changes in DSM-5 attempt to address, is the importance in distinguishing between intrusive memories and ruminative recollections of a traumatic event. Intrusive memories are experienced as unwanted and as clearly intruding into one's awareness, often out of the blue. Ruminations are more depressive thoughts that are consciously focused on and revisited. A failure to distinguish between these could lead to overdiagnosis of PTSD. Flashbacks are distinguished from intrusive memories or rumination by their dissociative quality. A flashback is not a strong memory; it is the subjective experience that the event is reoccurring in the present. Patients may report images, smells, or sounds from the event; may act out trauma-related behaviors; and may have complete amnesia for the episode. A less intense flashback may be described as feeling like a daydream and may include momentary loss of orientation to place. Assessment and diagnosis should include direct questions about symptoms, and interviewers should ask for specific examples to determine whether a diagnostic criterion is met.

An error that could lead to underdiagnosis is the assumption that nightmares experienced in PTSD must have an overt and obvious link to the trauma—that they are a replaying of the details of the event. However, DSM-5 specifies that trauma-related nightmares may reflect traumatic related affect rather than the exact details of the traumatic incident itself. For example, among many patients, nightmares are described as having thematic content, often a specific emotional theme such as threat, powerlessness, or intense fear that is reflective of the patients' subjective experience of trauma. For patients with multiple traumas, this may be particularly true.

COMORBID DISORDERS

Eighty percent of patients with PTSD have comorbid psychiatric disorders, and these patients also have high rates of medical comorbidities (Kessler et al. 1995). The most common psychiatric comorbidities include major depressive disorder, panic disorder, and substance use disorders. As noted earlier in the section "Biology," patients with PTSD also have high rates of diseases associated with increased allostatic load and inflammatory processes, including diiabetes, obesity, and autoimmune, cardiovascular, and gastrointestinal diseases (Boscarino 2004; Qureshi et al. 2009). Patients with PTSD also have higher mortality rates than individuals without PTSD (Boscarino 2006). Patients with PTSD are among the highest primary care users, and management may involve coordination with primary care or specialist providers treating comorbid somatic or medical complaints (Chan et al. 2009). PTSD is also associated with increased rates of sexual dysfunction and loss of sexual interest, even among relatively young patients and regardless of the nature of the trauma (Yehuda et al. 2015). Side-effect profiles of potential pharmacotherapies should be carefully considered and discussed with patients in light of medical problems.

Psychotherapies for comorbid psychiatric conditions may be integrated (treated by the same provider), sequential, or concurrent (treated separately but during the same period). Treatment of a primary disorder may result in remission across disorders. For example, trauma-focused therapy alone has been associated with reductions in depression and panic symptoms. Decisions about care should be made on an individual basis with consideration of symptom severity, the relationships among the conditions, acute safety or harm reduction, patient preference, and availability of services. Although integrated treatment is generally supported, research on treatment of comorbid conditions is preliminary, and evidence-based guidelines remain to be established.

DIFFERENTIAL DIAGNOSIS

Given the number of symptoms and symptom combinations that are possible when an individual meets criteria for PTSD, there are a number of other disorders that frequently must be ruled out. Mood disorders share many symptoms with PTSD, but there are some key issues for consideration. For example, major depressive episodes may occur in the aftermath of trauma but do not specifically include reexperiencing symptoms such as nightmares, intrusive memories, or efforts to avoid reminders of the trauma. In addition, the irritability associated with PTSD is usually variable and reactive (rather than pervasive and consistent as in mania). Finally, the sleep disruption in PTSD does not reflect a reduced need for sleep (although nightmares may lead to a reduced desire for sleep), and the impulsiveness is not linked specifically to periods of mood elevation and irritability.

Challenges may also arise when trying to differentiate between chronic PTSD and some personality disorders, particularly borderline personality disorder and antisocial personality disorder. For example, individuals with PTSD often exhibit behaviors and symptoms consistent with borderline personality disorder, such as chronic emotional dysregulation or interpersonal and behavioral problems. In some cases, absence of a Criterion A trauma can provide diagnostic clarity—in personality disorder there is no requirement for a specific antecedent, although patients with personality disorder frequently report childhood trauma. Indeed, there has been a debate in the literature, noted earlier (see section "Diagnostic Criteria"), regarding the construct of complex PTSD as a chronic syndrome that develops in response to prolonged or intense interpersonal trauma, usually in childhood. Where childhood trauma does exist, the clinician's ability to link the behavioral and emotional responses to trauma-related changes in worldview and sense of self may be relevant in determining whether the presentation is more consistent with PTSD.

Although PTSD is no longer classified among the anxiety disorders in DSM-5, anxious mood, fear-related avoidance, and panic attacks are all common among PTSD sufferers. It is therefore important to clarify the source or focus of the anxiety to differentiate symptoms of PTSD from those of anxiety disorders. For example, many individuals with PTSD engage in apparently compulsive behaviors such as repeated checking of doors and windows; this is commonly thought of as one aspect of the exaggerated concerns for safety and hypervigilance characteristic of the disorder. Other behaviors such as repeated washing may reflect the experience of being physically violated rather than a delusional concern with cleanliness. Unwanted intrusive thoughts are distinguished from obsessions in that they are related to the trauma and are not irrational in content. Phobic avoidance can usually be distinguished from the avoidance of trauma-related cues and reminders in PTSD; in phobias the avoidance is normally driven by fear of the cue. Panic attacks in PTSD tend to be triggered by trauma-related reminders or cues and do not occur unprovoked as in panic disorder. In addition, the agoraphobic avoidance in panic disorder is focused on avoiding a panic attack rather than the distress associated with a trauma-related reminder. Finally, pervasive worry in PTSD is focused on safety- or trauma-related concerns rather than the global "everyday" worries that tend to be associated with generalized anxiety disorder. This differentiation is shown to be important in the following case vignette.

Case Vignette

Ms. N, a 25-year-old white female, presented to treatment with complaints of depressed mood, anxiety, and difficulty concentrating. She attributed these problems to adjustment to college life and to the challenges of having moved to a large metropolitan city and losing her support network. She described periods of depression in the past and a history of being treated for ADHD and anxiety as a preteen when her parents divorced. At intake she denied exposure to trauma and was given diagnoses of major depressive disorder, rule-out generalized anxiety disorder. During the first month of psychotherapy, Ms. N also reported concerns about her alcohol consumption and described drinking with her college friends in a manner that led to impulsive behavior (emotional reactivity or sexual encounters) about which she was subsequently uncomfortable. As the presentation became more complicated, the intake information was reviewed again with the patient, and, now in the context of a developing alliance, Ms. N acknowledged that she had witnessed her mother attempt suicide when she was 5 years old. She completed the PCL-5, on which she scored 38. Diagnostic assessment then identified that the patient did meet criteria for PTSD.

EARLY INTERVENTION

Although PTSD is not diagnosed until clinically distressing or impairing symptoms have persisted longer than 1 month, acute stress disorder (ASD) may be diagnosed 3 days following exposure to a Criterion A trauma when there are nine or more symptoms from any of the four PTSD symptom clusters described in the earlier section "Diagnostic Criteria." There has been significant interest in early interventions for acutely traumatized patients to help manage symptoms and prevent the development of PTSD. Early responses should include psychoeducation, normalization of responses through education regarding common reactions to trauma, and ensuring that basic needs are being met. For individuals who do not meet ASD diagnostic criteria, ongoing monitoring, including the use of validated screening tools (see earlier section "Assessment and Diagnosis"), is recommended.

There is evidence for the efficacy of brief (four to five sessions) cognitive-behavioral therapy (CBT) for patients with ASD or significant symptoms, commencing at least 2 weeks after the trauma (Litz et al. 2002). Such therapy includes psychoeducation, relaxation, imaginal and in vivo exposure, and cognitive restructuring. Psychotherapy for individuals not reporting symptoms is not recommended and may even be harmful. Similarly, individual psychological debriefing, an umbrella term for interventions that involve a single session within a month of trauma exposure and include recollection of thoughts and emotions during the traumatic event, has been found to be ineffective and potentially harmful. No pharmacological treatments have been found to prevent ASD or PTSD, but medications may be used for the management of symptoms such as sleep disturbance, hyperarousal, and pain. There is some evidence that the administration of cortisol in the acute aftermath of trauma may have a prophylactic effect, but studies are ongoing and there is currently insufficient evidence to support this intervention (Steckler and Risbrough 2012).

TREATMENT GUIDELINES

Therapies for PTSD include evidence-based psychotherapies and pharmacotherapy, as well as adjunctive or supplemental interventions. Current research supports the use of either psychotherapy or pharmacotherapy as a first-line treatment; there is no clear evidence for the superiority of a combined approach. Clinical studies demonstrate strong support for the efficacy of specialized trauma-focused psychotherapy (described in the following subsection, "Psychotherapy"), although response rates are lower for combat veterans (Foa et al. 2008; Powers et al. 2010; U.S. Department of Veterans Affairs/Department of Defense 2010). Some patients, however, are not willing to engage in trauma-focused psychotherapy because of the distress associated with the process of treatment. In published pharmaceutical randomized clinical controlled trials, selective serotonin reuptake inhibitors (SSRIs) have been the most widely studied medications and have proven efficacy in reducing PTSD symptoms, with an approximate response rate of 60% (Bisson and Andrew 2009). Providers should discuss all treatment options, including potential side effects and the time commitment. Treatment guidelines for PTSD have been published by both the International Society for Traumatic Stress Studies (ISTSS) and the U.S. Department of Veterans Affairs/Department of Defense (see Web sites listed in "Suggested Readings and Web Sites" at the end of this chapter); summaries of current clinical guidelines appear in the following subsections.

Psychotherapy

Trauma-focused therapies and stress inoculation training have the strongest evidence of effectiveness for reducing or eliminating PTSD symptoms. Trauma-focused therapies generally include exposure to trauma memories and/or cognitive restructuring, stress and anxiety management techniques, and psychoeducation about PTSD. The most widely researched and strongly supported therapies are prolonged exposure therapy (Foa et al. 2007), cognitive processing therapy (Resick and Schnicke 1993), and eye movement desensitization and reprocessing (EMDR; Shapiro and Solomon 1995). These manualized treatments are structured and time limited. Exposure therapies, such as prolonged exposure, involve a revisiting of the traumatic memory through repeated imaginal exposure (e.g., retelling the story of the trauma) or written or oral narratives. Cognitive therapies, such as cognitive processing therapy, emphasize identifying core beliefs, problematic thought patterns, and "stuck points," which are addressed through cognitive restructuring. Cognitive restructuring involves a process of Socratic questioning and remediation strategies in which the patient's trauma-related beliefs about self, others, and the world are challenged. EMDR similarly includes exposure and cognitive approaches, combined with eye movements (following a clinician's moving finger in the patient's visual field). It is unclear whether the eye movement component of EMDR is an essential mechanism of the treatment's effectiveness. Stress inoculation training (Meichenbaum and Cameron 1989), a form of CBT, does not include an explicit focus on the trauma but addresses PTSD symptoms such as avoidance, anxiety, and trauma-related cognitions. Other manualized, exposure-based therapies include narrative exposure therapy (Schauer et al. 2011), in which participants narrate their life story, focusing in detail on experiences of trauma, and brief eclectic psychotherapy (Gersons et al. 2004), which blends exposure elements with psychodynamic elements such as focus on the patient-therapist relationship and emphasis on shame and guilt.

Nightmares and sleep disturbance are a frequent complaint in PTSD. In addition to education regarding sleep hygiene, imagery rehearsal therapy (Krakow and Zadra 2006) and CBT for insomnia (Edinger and Carney 2014) have shown promising initial findings.

The following case vignette demonstrates use of psychotherapy for a patient with PTSD.

Case Vignette

Ms. R, a 30-year-old Hispanic female, sought treatment for depressed mood, panic attacks, and poor sleep. At intake she identified a history of having been raped once as a teenager but noted that she had subsequently returned to school, completed college and graduate school, and married and that her symptoms had begun only after she and her husband adopted a child. Assessment indicated that she met criteria for PTSD and major depressive disorder with moderate to severe symptoms of both (her PCL-5 score was 72). It was also determined that the panic attacks she experienced were all initially triggered by reminders of being assaulted but began to occur spontaneously and unprompted. Her avoidance of situations was now most commonly motivated by a fear of having a panic attack, and she was given an additional diagnosis of panic disorder.

Collaborative treatment planning was undertaken, and Ms. R and the therapist decided to focus treatment on reducing the frequency of the panic attacks first because they were occurring daily. She declined all psychopharmacological intervention. CBT for panic disorder was therefore initiated, and the patient began to experience a reduction in the frequency of her panic attacks within 3 weeks. Her treatment adherence (both attending sessions and completing homework assignments) then abruptly became sporadic. After about 6 weeks of this behavior, Ms. R admitted in treatment that there had been a second sexual assault that occurred recently and that she had not disclosed this incident to her husband. Following a couple of weeks of processing this disclosure (and a subsequent further drop in the frequency of panic attacks to one or two weekly), she embarked on a course of cognitive processing therapy, which she subsequently completed on a weekly schedule of 12 sessions. At completion of this therapy, she no longer met diagnostic criteria for PTSD (her PCL-5 score was 28), major depressive disorder, or panic disorder, and she decided to terminate from treatment having met her treatment goals.

Pharmacotherapy

Antidepressants, in particular SSRIs and serotonin-norepinephrine reuptake inhibitors (SNRIs), have proved effective in treating PTSD and are considered a first-line treatment, although no single antidepressant has been found to reliably result in remission of symptoms (Friedman et al. 2009). Sertraline and paroxetine are the only drugs approved by the U.S. Food and Drug Administration for treatment of PTSD; fluoxetine has also shown good results. The SNRI venlafaxine has also shown positive results in two trials (Friedman et al. 2009). Tricyclic antidepressants, mirtazapine, nefazodone, amitriptyline and imipramine, and monoamine oxidase inhibitors (phenelzine) have all been associated with global improvements in PTSD (specifically reexperiencing and hyperarousal symptoms) and are recommended for treatment of PTSD (U.S. Department of Veterans Affairs/Department of Defense 2010).

Although benzodiazepines are widely used for anxiety and panic, there is no evidence of their effectiveness in treating PTSD, and benzodiazepine use may worsen symptoms and impede recovery (U.S. Department of Veterans Affairs/ Department of Defense 2010). Benzodiazepine use is therefore not recommended in treating PTSD. High rates of comorbidity with substance use disorders provide additional reason to avoid benzodiazepine use in patients with PTSD. Guanfacine and anticonvulsants (tiagabine, topiramate, or valproate) have not demonstrated efficacy in treating PTSD and are also not recommended (U.S. Department of Veterans Affairs/Department of Defense 2010). Current research also does not support the use of bupropion, buspirone, trazodone, anticonvulsants (lamotrigine or gabapentin), or atypical antipsychotics for PTSD (U.S. Department of Veterans Affairs/Department of Defense 2010). Monotherapy should be optimized (maximize dose, allow 8-week response time) prior to change in drug or addition of new medication. PTSD is chronic for many patients, and responders may need to continue medication indefinitely, with periodic reassessment. One limitation of pharmacotherapy is the likelihood of relapse following discontinuation of medication, and such risk should be considered in conjunction with possible side effects when making treatment decisions (Friedman et al. 2009).

In terms of adjunctive therapy, the antihypertensive prazosin has been effective in reducing nightmares and improving sleep in at least five small studies (U.S. Department of Veterans Affairs/Department of Defense 2010). Risperidone has shown no adjunctive benefit, and there is inadequate evidence to support the addition of other atypical antipsychotics, sympatholytics, or anticonvulsants (U.S. Department of Veterans Affairs/Department of Defense 2010). Insomnia and sleep disturbance are frequent complaints in PTSD and become chronic for many patients. Sleep problems may be exacerbated by comorbid conditions such as pain, depression, and substance use or abuse. It is important to assess whether the patient is avoiding sleep or having significantly interrupted sleep due to disturbing nightmares, in which case prazosin may be beneficial. Overall, nonpharmacological interventions have equal or better short- and long-term outcomes for insomnia and sleep disturbance in PTSD than hypnotics alone or in combination with behavioral strategies (U.S. Department of Veterans Affairs/Department of Defense 2010). Trazodone may be helpful and may supplement antidepressant action. Hypnotics are considered a second-line intervention and should be used for only a brief period. Newer nonbenzodiazepine hypnotics, such as zolpidem, eszopiclone, and ramelteon, have shorter half-lives and lower risk of dependency (U.S. Department of Veterans Affairs/Department of Defense 2010). Patients should be educated regarding possible side effects and risks of dependency.

The following case vignette demonstrates use of combined pharmacotherapy and psychotherapy for a patient with PTSD.

Case Vignette

Mr. V, a 34-year-old African American combat veteran, presented to treatment complaining of anger and relationship problems. He reported that his wife insisted that he come to treatment because of his extreme emotional detachment from the family. His PCL-5 score was 68. After the PTSD diagnosis was confirmed, sertraline 25 mg/day was introduced and titrated upward over 4 weeks to 150 mg/day. Mr. V continued to report poor sleep and nightly nightmares, so trazodone 50 mg/day and prazosin 2 mg/day were introduced and subsequently increased to 100 mg/day and 6 mg/day, respectively. Mr. V noted reduced frequency of nightmares but no improvements in sleep, so trazodone was discontinued and zolpidem 5 mg/day was introduced and subsequently increased to 10 mg/day with some moderate improvements (5 hours of sleep per night reported). At this point his PCL score was 60. Trauma-focused psychotherapy options were introduced, and the next 6 weeks focused on increasing Mr. V's coping skills and enhancing his motivation to undergo prolonged exposure treatment. It took 16 weeks to complete prolonged exposure because the patient began avoiding sessions, but ultimately he did return, and after 12 sessions his PCL-5 score plateaued at 36. Mr. V continued to report hypervigilance, poor sleep (5–6 hours per night), irritability, and emotional detachment with much less frequent reexperiencing symptoms. His prazosin was discontinued and he was titrated off sertraline. Mr. V continued with psychotherapy to address residual symptoms.

CONCLUSION

PTSD is a significant mental health concern that affects approximately 7% of adults in the United States (Kessler et al. 2005). However, most people who are exposed to a traumatic experience recover; less than 25% develop PTSD (Riggs et al. 1995; Rothbaum et al. 1992). Recovery trajectories include resilience following trauma, recovery over time, and chronic PTSD. Risk for development of the disorder is compounded by the chronicity and severity of the trauma exposure, a personal or family history of mental illness, lack of posttrauma social support, female gender, and low intelligence and socioeconomic status, among other factors. PTSD can be a debilitating disorder with significant functional impairment and a damaging effect on family and intimate relationships. Patients should be screened for trauma exposure and assessed for symptoms. For those with PTSD, education regarding common symptoms and treatment options is essential. Both trauma-focused psychotherapies and pharmacotherapy with SSRIs have demonstrated efficacy in treating PTSD, although many patients who experience symptom reduction continue to have clinically significant symptoms that require ongoing treatment.

Key Points

- Posttraumatic stress disorder (PTSD) occurs in approximately 15%–25% of those who experience trauma, with a population lifetime prevalence rate of 3.6% in men and 9.7% in women.

- Multiple posttrauma trajectories have been identified, and these vary somewhat by study and population. The majority of people demonstrate resilience in the face of trauma and do not develop PTSD. Other trajectories include initial distress followed by recovery, chronic symptoms, and delayed onset of symptoms.

- Risk factors for PTSD include pretraumatic, peritraumatic, and posttraumatic factors. These include female gender, prior trauma or adversity, severity of trauma, dissociation during the trauma, poor social support, and poor coping skills.

- PTSD has been associated with increased glucocorticoid sensitivity and prolonged sympathetic system activation, which increase the risk of comorbid medical conditions associated with chronic allostatic load and glucocorticoid function, including diabetes and obesity and autoimmune, cardiovascular, and gastrointestinal diseases.

- PTSD has high rates (approximately 80%) of psychiatric comorbidities, including major depressive disorder, panic disorder, and substance use disorders, which are important to consider in differential diagnosis and are relevant for treatment planning.

- PTSD is not diagnosed until 1 month after the trauma exposure, but in the case of significant symptoms persisting at least 2 weeks posttrauma, brief cognitive-behavioral therapy (four to five sessions) that includes exposure and/or cognitive restructuring may be effective in reducing symptoms and preventing PTSD.

- Current treatment guidelines support the use of psychotherapy and pharmacotherapy as first-line treatments; there is no clear evidence for the superiority of a combined approach.

- Among psychotherapeutic approaches, trauma-focused therapies and stress inoculation training have the strongest empirical support for efficacy. Trauma-focused therapies include exposure to trauma memories and/or cognitive restructuring, stress and anxiety management techniques, and psychoeducation. Stress inoculation training addresses PTSD symptoms such as avoidance, anxiety, and trauma-related cognitions.

- Antidepressants, in particular selective serotonin reuptake inhibitors, have proven effectiveness in treating PTSD and are considered a first-line treatment. Sertraline and paroxetine are the only drugs approved by the U.S. Food and Drug Administration for treatment of PTSD; fluoxetine has also shown good results.

- Benzodiazepines have been shown to have harmful effects and are discouraged in the treatment of PTSD.

SUGGESTED READINGS AND WEB SITES

Readings

Institute of Medicine: Treatment of Posttraumatic Stress Disorder: An Assessment of the Evidence. Washington, DC, National Academies Press, 2008

Ipser JC, Stein DJ: Evidence-based pharmacotherapy of post-traumatic stress disorder (PTSD). Int J Neuropsychopharmacol 15(6):825–840, 2012 21798109

Watts BV, Schnurr PP, Mayo L, et al: Meta-analysis of the efficacy of treatments for post-traumatic stress disorder. J Clin Psychiatry 74(6):e541–e550, 2013 23842024

Web Sites

International Society for Traumatic Stress Studies (ISTSS): www.istss.org

National Center for PTSD: www.ptsd.va.gov

National Institute of Mental Health: www.nimh.nih.gov/health/topics/post-traumatic-stress-disorder-ptsd

TREATMENT GUIDELINES

International Society for Traumatic Stress Studies Treatment Guidelines: www.istss.org/treating-trauma/effective-treatments-for-ptsd,-2nd-edition.aspx

U.S. Department of Veterans Affairs/Department of Defense Clinical Practice Guidelines: www.healthquality.va.gov/guidelines/MH/ptsd/

REFERENCES

American Psychiatric Association: Diagnostic and Statistical Manual of Mental Disorders, 3rd Edition. Washington, DC, American Psychiatric Association, 1980

American Psychiatric Association: Diagnostic and Statistical Manual of Mental Disorders, 4th Edition. Washington, DC, American Psychiatric Association, 1994

American Psychiatric Association: Diagnostic and Statistical Manual of Mental Disorders, 5th Edition. Arlington, VA, American Psychiatric Association, 2013

Amos T, Stein DJ, Ipser JC: Pharmacological interventions for preventing post-traumatic stress disorder (PTSD). Cochrane Database Syst Rev 7:CD006239, 2014 25001071

Bisson J, Andrew M: Psychological treatment of post-traumatic stress disorder (PTSD). Cochrane Database Syst Rev (3):CD003388, 2007 17636720

Boscarino JA: Posttraumatic stress disorder and physical illness: results from clinical and epidemiologic studies. Ann NY Acad Sci 1032(1):141–153, 2004 15677401

Boscarino JA: Posttraumatic stress disorder and mortality among U.S. Army veterans 30 years after military service. Ann Epidemiol 16(4):248–256, 2006 16099672

Brewin CR, Andrews B, Valentine JD: Meta-analysis of risk factors for posttraumatic stress disorder in trauma-exposed adults. J Consult Clin Psychol 68(5):748–766, 2000 11068961

Chan D, Cheadle AD, Reiber G, et al: Health care utilization and its costs for depressed veterans with and without comorbid PTSD symptoms. Psychiatr Serv 60(12):1612–1617, 2009 19952151

Cloitre M, Petkova E, Wang J, et al: An examination of the influence of a sequential treatment on the course and impact of dissociation among women with PTSD related to childhood abuse. Depress Anxiety 29(8):709–717, 2012 22550033

Daskalakis NP, Lehrner A, Yehuda R: Endocrine aspects of post-traumatic stress disorder and implications for diagnosis and treatment. Endocrinol Metab Clin North Am 42(3):503–513, 2013 24011883

Edinger JD, Carney CE: Overcoming Insomnia: A Cognitive-Behavioral Therapy Approach, Therapist Guide. New York, Oxford University Press, 2014

Foa E, Hembree E, Rothbaum BO: Prolonged Exposure Therapy for PTSD: Emotional Processing of Traumatic Experiences, Therapist Guide. New York, Oxford University Press, 2007

Foa EB, Keane TM, Friedman MJ: Effective Treatments for PTSD: Practice Guidelines From the International Society for Traumatic Stress Studies. New York, Guilford, 2008

Friedman MJ, Davidson JRT, Stein DJ: Psychopharmacotherapy for adults, in Effective Treatments for PTSD: Practice Guidelines from the International Society for Traumatic Stress Studies. Edited by Foa EB, Keane TM, Friedman MJ, et al. New York, Guilford, 2009, pp 245–268

Friedman MJ, Resick PA, Bryant RA, et al: Considering PTSD for DSM-5. Depress Anxiety 28(9):750–769, 2011 21910184

Gersons B, Carlier I, Olff M: Manual Brief Eclectic Psychotherapy (BEP) for Posttraumatic Stress Disorder. Amsterdam, Academic Medical Centre, 2004

Herman JL: Complex PTSD: A syndrome in survivors of prolonged and repeated trauma. J Trauma Stress 5(3):377–391, 1992

Kessler RC, Sonnega A, Bromet E, et al: Posttraumatic stress disorder in the National Comorbidity Survey. Arch Gen Psychiatry 52:1048–1060, 1995

Kessler RC, Berglund P, Demler O, et al: Lifetime prevalence and age-of-onset distributions of DSM-IV disorders in the National Comorbidity Survey Replication. Arch Gen Psychiatry 62(6):593–602, 2005 15939837

Krakow B, Zadra A: Clinical management of chronic nightmares: imagery rehearsal therapy. Behav Sleep Med 4(1):45–70, 2006 16390284

Lanius RA, Brand B, Vermetten E, et al: The dissociative subtype of posttraumatic stress disorder: rationale, clinical and neurobiological evidence, and implications. Depress Anxiety 29(8):701–708, 2012 22431063

Litz BT, Gray MJ, Bryant RA, et al: Early intervention for trauma: current status and future directions. Clin Psychol Sci Pract 9(2):112–134, 2002

Meichenbaum D, Cameron R: Stress Inoculation Training. New York, Springer, 1989

National Comorbidity Survey: NCS-R appendix tables. National Comorbidity Survey, 2005. Available at: www.hcp.med.harvard.edu/ncs/publications.php. Accessed September 9, 2015.

Neylan TC, Schadt EE, Yehuda R: Biomarkers for combat-related PTSD: focus on molecular networks from high-dimensional data. Eur J Psychotraumatol 5: 2014 25206954

Ozer EJ, Best SR, Lipsey TL, et al: Predictors of posttraumatic stress disorder and symptoms in adults: a meta-analysis. Psychol Bull 129(1):52–73, 2003 12555794

Pietrzak RH, Feder A, Singh R, et al: Trajectories of PTSD risk and resilience in World Trade Center responders: an 8-year prospective cohort study. Psychol Med 44(1):205–219, 2014 23551932

Pitman RK, Rasmusson AM, Koenen KC, et al: Biological studies of post-traumatic stress disorder. Nat Rev Neurosci 13(11):769–787, 2012 23047775

Powers MB, Halpern JM, Ferenschak MP, et al: A meta-analytic review of prolonged exposure for posttraumatic stress disorder. Clin Psychol Rev 30(6)635–641, 2010 20546985

Pratchett LC, Pelcovitz MR, Yehuda R: Trauma and violence: are women the weaker sex? Psychiatr Clin North Am 33(2):465–474, 2010 20385347

Qureshi SU, Pyne JM, Magruder KM, et al: The link between post-traumatic stress disorder and physical comorbidities: a systematic review. Psychiatr Q 80(2):87–97, 2009 19291401

Resick PA, Schnicke M: Cognitive Processing Therapy for Rape Victims: A Treatment Manual, Vol 4. New York, Sage, 1993

Resick PA, Suvak MK, Johnides BD, et al: The impact of dissociation on PTSD treatment with cognitive processing therapy. Depress Anxiety 29(8):718–730, 2012 22473922

Riggs DS, Rothbaum BO, Foa EB: Prospective examination of symptoms of posttraumatic stress disorder in victims of nonsexual assault. J Interpers Violence 10(2):201–214, 1995

Rothbaum BO, Foa EB, Riggs DS, et al: A prospective examination of post-traumatic stress disorder in rape victims. J Trauma Stress 5(3):455–475, 1992

Schauer M, Neuner F, Elbert T: Narrative Exposure Therapy: A Short-Term Intervention for Traumatic Stress Disorders, 2nd Edition. Cambridge, MA, Hogrefe, 2011

Shapiro F, Solomon RM: Eye Movement Desensitization and Reprocessing: Basic Principles, Protocols, and Procedures New York, Guilford, 1995

Shin LM, Liberzon I: The neurocircuitry of fear, stress, and anxiety disorders. Neuropsychopharmacology 35(1):169–191, 2010 19625997

Steckler T, Risbrough V: Pharmacological treatment of PTSD—established and new approaches. Neuropharmacology 62(2):617–627, 2012 21736888

Stein DJ, Koenen KC, Friedman MJ, et al: Dissociation in posttraumatic stress disorder: evidence from the World Mental Health Surveys. Biol Psychiatry 73(4):302–312, 2013 23059051

U.S. Department of Veterans Affairs/Department of Defense: VA/DoD Clinical Practice Guideline for Management of Post-Traumatic Stress. Washington, DC, U.S. Department of Veterans Affairs/Department of Defense, 2005. Available at: www.healthquality.va.gov/guidelines/MH/ptsd/. Accessed September 9, 2015.

van Zuiden M, Kavelaars A, Geuze E, et al: Predicting PTSD: pre-existing vulnerabilities in glucocorticoid-signaling and implications for preventive interventions. Brain Behav Immun 30:12–21, 2013 22981834

Weathers FW, Litz BT, Keane TM, et al: The PTSD Checklist for DSM-5 (PCL-5). Washington, DC, National Center for PTSD, U.S. Department of Veterans Affairs. 2013. Available at: www.ptsd.va.gov. Accessed September 9, 2015.

Wolf EJ, Miller MW, Reardon AF, et al: A latent class analysis of dissociation and posttraumatic stress disorder: evidence for a dissociative subtype. Arch Gen Psychiatry 69(7):698–705, 2012 22752235

Yehuda R: Status of glucocorticoid alterations in post-traumatic stress disorder. Ann N Y Acad Sci 1179:56–69, 2009 19906232

Yehuda R, McFarlane AC: Conflict between current knowledge about posttraumatic stress disorder and its original conceptual basis. Am J Psychiatry 152(12):1705–1713, 1995 8526234

Yehuda R, Lehrner A, Rosenbaum TY: PTSD and sexual dysfunction in men and women. J Sex Med 12(5):1107–1119, 2015 25847589

Zoladz PR, Diamond DM: Current status on behavioral and biological markers of PTSD: a search for clarity in a conflicting literature. Neurosci Biobehav Rev 37(5):860–895, 2013 23567521

CHAPTER 7

Disintegrated Experience

DISSOCIATION AND STRESS

DAVID SPIEGEL, M.D.

PSYCHIATRISTS AND psychologists have been divided about dissociation since the earliest days of these professions. The pioneering psychologist Pierre Janet (1889) usefully described dissociation as *desaggregation mentale,* a means of managing emotional conflict by isolating memory, usually involving traumatic experience, from current cognition and affect. Sigmund Freud, a psychiatrist by training. linked the limitations of consciousness to early-life trauma (Breuer and Freud 1893–1895/1955), a point of view he later revised to emphasize primitive unconscious sexual desire rather than traumatic experience. For both Janet and Freud, dissociation was an early and obvious model of unconscious mental processing, as well as a type of psychopathology. Freud used hypnosis, a form of controlled dissociation, in his early treatment of what was then called hysteria. The link between hypnosis and dissociation has led to much research on the ability to separate and unite elements of consciousness (Hilgard 1977). Despite, or perhaps because of, this redoubtable history and substantial evidence linking trauma and dissociation (Dalenberg et al. 2012), some still consider dissociation a "sideshow" rather than a legitimate mental disorder—that is, a drama induced by credulous therapists rather than an expression of distress often linked to trauma. Dissociative disorders occur around the world (Spiegel et al. 2011), and it should not be surprising that with mood and anxiety disorders involving uncontrolled fluctuation in affect and schizophrenia demonstrating impaired cognition and disconnection from af-

119

fect, there would plausibly exist mental disorders that occur because of a failure to adequately integrate and control elements of consciousness and affect. A person's experience of mental unity is an achievement, not a given, and it is most profoundly challenged by traumatic discontinuities in experience.

NEUROBIOLOGY UNDERLYING DISSOCIATIVE SYMPTOMATOLOGY

Traumatic experience imposes strong cognitive and affective processing demands because memories of the experience are associated with strong emotional valence. This has most commonly been acknowledged with a fear-based model of posttraumatic stress disorder (PTSD), with intrusion and hyperarousal alternating with avoidance. However, dissociation is a different response to trauma, involving inhibition rather than activation. Research has been conducted on the neuronal underpinnings of reexperiencing, hyperarousal, and depersonalization/derealization dissociative responses in PTSD using a script-driven symptom provocation paradigm (Lanius et al. 2006). In this paradigm the patient creates a narrative of his or her traumatic experience with as many sensory details as possible. These narratives are then read back to the patient, who is instructed to recall the traumatic memory as vividly as possible, during functional magnetic resonance imaging. Responses to this same condition are of two types. Approximately 70% of patients demonstrate undermodulation, reexperiencing the trauma with limbic activation and a concomitant increase in heart rate. Another 30%, however, exhibit states of depersonalization and derealization, limbic inhibition, and no significant concomitant increase in heart rate (Lanius et al. 2010). This latter group demonstrates overmodulation rather than undermodulation of their affective response to trauma memories.

Emotional Undermodulation: Failure of Corticolimbic Inhibition

Emotional undermodulation can be identified by symptoms of reexperiencing and hyperarousal typical of the intrusion cluster of PTSD symptoms. Those who respond to hearing their trauma narratives with reexperiencing and hyperarousal symptoms exhibit abnormally *low* activation in the medial prefrontal and the anterior cingulate cortex. These brain regions play a crucial role in modulating arousal and regulating emotion (Etkin and Wager 2007; Lanius et al. 2006). Neuroimaging investigations in patients with PTSD have clearly demonstrated inhibitory influence of the prefrontal cortex on the amygdala. Consistent with impaired cortical modulation of affect and arousal, increased activation of the limbic system, particularly the amygdala, has often been demonstrated in patients with PTSD in response to exposure to traumatic reminders and to masked fearful faces (Etkin and Wager 2007). Positron emission tomography studies of individuals with PTSD have shown a negative correlation between blood flow in the left ventromedial prefrontal cortex and the amygdala, as well as a negative correlation between medial prefrontal cortex and the amygdala during exposure to fearful faces (Shin et al. 2005). *Decreased* activation of medial prefrontal regions observed in the reexperiencing/hyperaroused PTSD subgroup is therefore consistent with failed inhibition of limbic and especially amygdala reactivity and is associated with reexperiencing/hyperaroused emotional undermodulation (Francati et al. 2007).

Emotional Overmodulation: Excessive Corticolimbic Inhibition

Emotional overmodulation characterizes dissociative symptoms, including depersonalization and derealization, which usually involve distancing from an emotional experience. In contrast to the reexperiencing/hyperaroused group described in the previous subsection, those experiencing symptoms of depersonalization and derealization exhibit abnormally *high* activation in the anterior cingulate cortex and the medial prefrontal cortex and concomitant hyperinhibition of limbic regions, including the amygdala (Lanius et al. 2006, 2010). Dissociation in the immediate aftermath of trauma is associated with activation of occipital and parahippocampal regions involved in traumatic memory of emotional events, leading later to intrusive recollection (Daniels et al. 2012).

An investigation by Felmingham et al. (2008) provides further evidence for the corticolimbic inhibition model of dissociation. This study compared brain activation patterns during the processing of consciously and nonconsciously perceived fear stimuli. PTSD patients with high state-dissociation scores during the neuroimaging procedure, as measured by the Clinician Administered Dissociative States Scale (CADSS), showed enhanced activation in the ventral prefrontal cortex during conscious fear processing when compared with patients with low state-dissociation scores. During processing of nonconscious fear, high dissociative symptomatology at the time of the scan was associated with increased activation in the bilateral amygdala, insula, and left thalamus, as compared with low state dissociation. The authors propose that dissociation, including states of depersonalization and derealization, is an emotion-regulatory strategy during conscious processing of threat that is employed to cope with extreme arousal in PTSD through hyperinhibition of limbic regions. These findings indicate that dissociators are not incapable of emotional arousal and that what is kept out of sight is not out of mind.

DISSOCIATION IN DSM-5

Dissociative disorders have been described as a "disease of hiddenness" (Kluft 1991) because the symptoms involve amnesia and other interference with conscious awareness and because the disorders often result from traumatic experiences such as childhood abuse that involve shame and a protective need to hide. Thus, the very presence of these disorders, especially dissociative identity disorder, implies the possibility of mistreatment earlier in life, leading to inevitable disputes about the diagnosis. Although some argued that the dissociative disorders should disappear from DSM-5 (Paris 2012), the weight of the evidence led to their continued inclusion, in revised form (Spiegel et al. 2011). However, future changes are possible; the use of the Arabic rather than Roman numeral (DSM-5 rather than DSM-V) is meant to indicate that DSM is and will continue to be a work in progress, and updates will be numbered DSM-5.1, 5.2, and so on. The link between dissociation and trauma has been strengthened in DSM-5.

Dissociative Identity Disorder

The flagship diagnosis, dissociative identity disorder, remains, with its emphasis on disruption of identity characterized by "the presence of two or more distinct personality states or an experience of possession" (American Psychiatric Association 2013, p. 291). The addition of possession allows inclusion of types of pathological dissociation that occur in non-Western cultures as well as minority cultures in the West. The definition of dissociative identity disorder has also been altered to emphasize the intrusive nature of the dissociative symptoms as disruptions in consciousness. The diagnostic criteria have also been extended to include mention of the fact that dissociative amnesia often occurs for everyday as well as traumatic events.

Dissociative Amnesia

Dissociative amnesia is described as "an inability to recall important autobiographical information, usually of a traumatic or stressful nature" (American Psychiatric Association 2013, p. 298). The rarer form involving more global amnesia for identity associated with "purposeful travel or bewildered wandering," which was associated in DSM-IV with a diagnosis of dissociative fugue (American Psychiatric Association 1994), is now diagnosed using a specifier, "with dissociative fugue." This change is largely because fugue is very rare, is almost uniformly associated with amnesia, and does not always involve aimless wandering (Spiegel et al. 2011, 2013).

Case Vignette

A married man with a responsible job as a civil engineer had an accident in which he suffered a serious electrical shock from a high-voltage source. His physical injuries healed, but he became boyish and insisted that his wife was his mother and had to take care of him. He could not remember any work-related skills. Looking at the computer on my desk he asked, "Why is that television attached to a typewriter?" The patient had no evidence of head trauma or central neurological injury, and a diagnosis of dissociative amnesia with dissociative fugue was made.

Depersonalization Disorder

Depersonalization disorder has been renamed depersonalization/derealization disorder in DSM-5 because the symptoms of derealization frequently co-occur with persistent depersonalization (Spiegel et al. 2013). Although this disorder may occur without exposure to stressful or traumatic experiences, evidence has accumulated that depersonalization and derealization occur commonly during trauma and may accompany other PTSD symptoms as well (Spiegel et al. 2013).

Dissociative Subtype of PTSD

Another important change in DSM-5 underscoring the connection between trauma and dissociation is the introduction of a dissociative subtype of PTSD (Ginzburg et al. 2006; Spiegel et al. 2013). This change, which involves the addition of depersonalization/derealization symptoms to those required for PTSD, is expected to describe about 10%–15% of PTSD cases (Stein et al. 2013). It is the result of research demonstrating different phenomenology from the more common intrusion and hyperarousal symptoms (Ginzburg et al. 2006; Waelde et al. 2005), although dissociative flashbacks are included among them. The neuroimaging research reviewed earlier (see "Neurobiology Underlying Dissociative Symptomatology") has provided empirical basis for this addition. Also, results from epidemiological, prevalence, and treatment studies, discussed in the following sections, provide further support for this DSM-5 change.

EPIDEMIOLOGICAL EVIDENCE

A recent epidemiological study involving 25,018 people from 16 countries in a World Health Organization World Mental Health Survey found that 14.4% of those with PTSD also had the dissociative symptoms of depersonalization and derealization (Stein et al. 2013). They were also characterized by higher levels of reexperiencing symptoms, onset of PTSD in childhood, high trauma exposure and childhood adversities, severe role impairment, and suicidality. Research suggests that dissociation is associated with unresponsive parenting and psychological trauma, as well as PTSD (e.g., Dalenberg et al. 2012; Ginzburg et al. 2006; Lanius et al. 2010, 2012; Wolf et al. 2012a, 2012b). Although not all individuals who meet criteria for PTSD have high levels of dissociation, most individuals with high levels of dissociative symptomatology meet criteria for PTSD.

PREVALENCE

Dissociative disorders are more common than usually thought. In a study by Waller and Ross (1997), 3% of the general population met criteria for a dissociative disorder. In other studies, 29% of an inner-city psychiatric outpatient population (Foote et al. 2006) and 9% of an adult day care population (Lussier et al. 1997) were found to have a dissociative disorder, in most cases associated with a history of sexual and physical abuse. Furthermore, individuals with dissociation differ in symptom profiles among traumatized individuals. In one study among 316 veterans, one-third of those who had PTSD had a distinct dissociative disorder subtype (Waelde et al. 2005).

SYMPTOM PROFILE

Wolf et al. (2012a, 2012b) used latent class analysis to examine PTSD and dissociative symptomatology in 492 veterans and their partners, not all of whom met criteria for PTSD. Of the individuals who did meet criteria for PTSD using the Clinician-Administered PTSD Scale (CAPS; Weathers et al. 2001), 12% formed a dissociative group characterized by high PTSD symptoms and elevated dissociation scores, specifically derealization and depersonalization, as well as significantly more flashbacks. Although the classic PTSD symptom clusters were strongly intercorrelated, they did not correlate as highly with the derealization or depersonalization items (both r=0.27, P<0.001). The authors further validated these findings using latent profile analyses on symptoms of PTSD and dissociation (depersonalization, derealization, and reduction in awareness of surroundings) among 360 male Vietnam War veterans with combat-related PTSD and 284 female veterans and active-duty service personnel with PTSD and a high base rate of exposure to sexual trauma. As in the first study by Wolf and colleagues (Wolf et al. 2012a), the latent profile analysis yielded evidence for a three-class solution in both samples, including moderate and high PTSD classes as well as a class marked by high PTSD severity coupled with dissociative symptoms, including depersonalization, derealization, and a reduction in awareness of surroundings.

    In the latter study (Wolf et al. 2012b), approximately 15% of the male sample and 30% of the female sample were classified into the dissociative subtype. Women (but not men) with the dissociative subtype of PTSD exhibited higher rates of DSM-IV Axis II comorbidity, including avoidant and borderline personality disorders. In a civilian PTSD sample consisting predominantly of women with histories of childhood trauma, evidence for a dissociative subtype of PTSD emerged using latent class and confirmatory factor analyses (Lanius et al. 2012). As in the studies by Wolf et al. (2012a, 2012b), latent class analysis yielded three groups, one of which was uniquely characterized by high derealization and depersonalization symptoms (and accounted for 25% of the sample). Individuals in this dissociative subgroup also had a higher number of comorbid Axis I disorders and a more significant history of childhood abuse and neglect. Furthermore, confirmatory factor analyses suggested a five-factor solution in which depersonalization and derealization symptoms are distinct from, but correlate significantly with, the core PTSD symptom clusters.

In addition to a history of childhood sexual and physical abuse, other factors associated later in life with dissociative symptoms include physical violence, shame, and guilt (Dorahy et al. 2013).

IMPLICATIONS FOR TREATMENT

As discussed in previous sections, neurobiological, epidemiological, and latent class analysis data provide support for a distinct subtype of PTSD involving dissociation. In addition, evidence suggests that high levels of dissociation appear to be associated with differential response to some conventional PTSD treatments. Findings from a study by Jaycox et al. (1998) suggested that dissociation during traumatic memory processing may interfere with habituation, a critical process for resolving PTSD during exposure-based treatments.

One open-trial study of prolonged exposure found that PTSD subjects who exhibited high-dissociative symptomatology were more likely to maintain their diagnosis of PTSD at the end of treatment (69%) than were those with low-dissociative symptomatology (10%), even though both groups showed equal improvement in PTSD symptoms posttreatment (Hagenaars et al. 2010). Several other impressive treatment trials (Cloitre et al. 2012; Resick et al. 2012) provide crucial evidence that identification of the dissociative subtype is not only descriptively but also clinically significant. Dissociative and hyperarousal subtypes of PTSD respond differently to treatment, and therefore better clinical outcome is linked to identification of the syndrome.

Cloitre, who has pioneered phase-oriented treatment of dissociative disorders, conducted a dismantling study in which three elements of psychotherapy—training in affect and relationship management, narrative storytelling, and supportive counseling—were employed. These three treatments were equally effective in reducing PTSD symptoms for patients low in dissociation, but for those with significant dissociative symptoms, the combination of skills

training and narrative storytelling provided better initial outcome, and supportive counseling helped to maintain posttreatment gains. Cloitre et al. (2012) randomly assigned women with childhood trauma–related PTSD to one of three
psychotherapeutic interventions. The treatment of principal interest included a
form of modified exposure therapy (labeled Narrative Story Telling, or NST)
preceded by a cognitive-behavioral intervention intended to facilitate the development of emotion regulation and interpersonal effectiveness skills (labeled
Skills Training in Affective and Interpersonal Regulation, or STAIR). This
STAIR/NST model was compared with two other forms of treatment delivery:
1) supportive counseling followed by NST and 2) STAIR followed by supportive
counseling. The STAIR/NST model had previously been shown to be the most
advantageous delivery model for most patients (Cloitre et al. 2010). A reanalysis
of the data, however, showed that among women reporting lower pretreatment
(baseline) levels of dissociative symptoms, outcomes across the three delivery
models in terms of dissociative symptoms were largely equivalent. However,
among women with high pretreatment levels of dissociation, dissociation was reduced most effectively by STAIR/NST; the effect was most obvious at 6-month
posttreatment follow-up. In addition, among those with higher posttreatment
dissociation scores, the greatest ongoing decreases in PTSD symptoms during
the course of follow-up occurred in the STAIR/NST group.

Similarly, Resick compared cognitive processing therapy to cognitive therapy
alone or written accounts about the trauma alone (Resick et al. 2008). She found
that high dissociators responded best to the combination of cognitive processing
and written accounts, whereas low dissociators responded to the cognitive processing without the addition of written accounts that documented sensory and
other aspects of the experience. Resick speculated that for high dissociators the
addition of writing may help them to identify and integrate disparate aspects of
their traumatic experience, whereas for low dissociators the writing may trigger
distressing associations to the trauma without helping to process them. Resick et
al. (2012) randomly assigned women with PTSD related to interpersonal violence
to one of three treatments: 1) cognitive therapy alone, 2) written exposure therapy
alone, or 3) cognitive processing therapy. The latter intervention combines elements of cognitive therapy and written exposure therapy. Outcomes were determined not only by PTSD symptoms but also by dissociative symptoms. Among
those women with high pretreatment baseline levels of dissociation, cognitive processing therapy achieved quicker and overall better outcomes on PTSD symptom
severity than did cognitive therapy alone, with outcomes for written exposure
therapy alone producing outcomes that did not significantly differ from either of
the two conditions. Importantly, group differences were observed only for certain
dissociation measures (Multiscale Dissociation Inventory depersonalization subscale but not Trauma Symptom Inventory dissociation subscale), suggesting the
need to examine different factors of dissociation on treatment outcome.

For PTSD with dissociation, the recommended treatment is complex and phase oriented and involves techniques designed to stabilize mood and teach emotion regulation in addition to working through trauma (Cloitre et al. 2011). These stabilization aspects are comparable to that used in dialectical behavior therapy for borderline personality disorder (Lanius and Tuhan 2003). Both studies show that treatment outcome can be improved by identifying dissociation.

Additional evidence for the influence of dissociation, including symptoms of depersonalization and derealization, on emotional learning stems from a study examining a classical conditioning paradigm to investigate the effects of state dissociation on acquisition and extinction processes in patients with borderline personality disorder (Ebner-Priemer et al. 2009). Individuals with borderline personality disorder and high levels of state dissociation did not show differences in skin conductance and arousal during acquisition and early extinction. In contrast, patients with borderline personality disorder and low levels of state dissociation (as well as healthy subjects) showed higher skin conductance and arousal during these processes. These findings, reminiscent of the observation of differences in heart rate reactivity to script-driven imagery reported by Lanius et al. (2006, 2010), suggest that emotional, amygdala-based learning processes are hindered by state dissociation, resulting in the alteration of acquisition and extinction processes. Ebner-Priemer et al. (2009) point out that dissociative patients should therefore be closely monitored in exposure-based psychotherapy because they may not respond to exposure treatment but rather may feel further traumatized. Those patients who have suffered abuse in childhood will expect that even well-meaning therapists will be inflicting further trauma rather than attempting to resolve posttraumatic symptomatology (i.e., "traumatic transference"). Exacerbation of problems such as comorbid depression and suicidality can be expected and must be monitored and managed. There are some patients with dissociative symptoms such as fugue who may not have a history of significant trauma but rather have life stressors such as complicated bereavement. Their amnesia for major components of their life history complicates psychotherapy. Techniques such as hypnosis can sometimes, but not always, help them to reorient.

There are no specific medications to treat these problems, although antidepressants, mood stabilizers, and antianxiety medications may play an adjunctive role, especially for comorbid disorders such as depression and anxiety. Furthermore, dissociation, including symptoms of depersonalization and derealization, has been demonstrated to be a negative predictor of psychotherapy outcome in patients with borderline personality disorder (Kleindienst et al. 2011).

Case Vignette

Ms. F, a 26-year-old woman, was seen in the emergency room for a deep self-inflicted knife wound in her thigh. She showed emotional lability and was alternately hostile and passive. She also had changes in memory with temporal disorientation.

At times she thought it was a year earlier and that she was in another hospital. She was admitted to the psychiatric inpatient unit and was initially diagnosed with borderline personality disorder and possible bipolar II disorder. She was started on antipsychotics, which did not improve her symptoms. Because of the possibility of fugue-like states, she was evaluated again, was found to be extremely hypnotizable, and was able to change temporal orientation in hypnosis. A further history of sexual abuse by a stepfather when Ms. F was 12 years old and of persistent changes in identity, including finding herself in places to which she could not remember going and being told she said things she did not remember, led to a diagnosis of dissociative identity disorder.

Intensive psychotherapy was instituted, including teaching Ms. F to use self-hypnosis to control access to different identity states and enhance communication across them. Once this ability to manage dissociation was established, the therapy turned to helping her work through memories of earlier sexual abuse by her drug-abusing stepfather. She was asked to focus on one element of the assault, using a split screen to picture it while maintaining in hypnosis a sense of comfort and safety in her body. She was then asked to picture one thing she had done to protect herself. She recalled one episode in which he forced her to have oral sex, but she then smiled and said, "I gagged and threw up all over him. He threw me against the wall, but I spoiled his fun." The therapy involved helping her to see the dissociation as a means of handling this history of trauma, including inappropriate self-blame for not avoiding the assaults. As she learned to control the dissociation and enhance understanding among these disparate identities, her symptoms receded. She was discharged from the hospital, continued in psychotherapy, and established her first relationship with a caring and nonabusive boyfriend.

CONCLUSION

The findings described in this chapter are consistent with the notion that dissociative symptoms can interfere with the cognitive and affective processing thought to mediate the efficacy of psychotherapy for PTSD (e.g., habituation, cognitive restructuring, emotion regulation). As a whole, these studies make it clear that trauma and dissociation are linked, that dissociation reflects the way brains function in response to trauma, and that awareness of this distinct subtype enhances treatment response.

Effective treatment of trauma-related dissociative disorders involves a primary focus on psychotherapy, with adjunctive use of medication for symptom control and treatment of comorbid disorders such as depression and anxiety. These are disorders of consciousness, often initially interrupted by stress and trauma. Salient psychotherapy includes attention to stabilization, emotion regulation, stress management, working through traumatic experiences, and consolidation of treatment gains. Psychiatry has focused on disrupted cognition (schizophrenia) and mood (depression, bipolar disorder) but has paid less attention to intrusions into and gaps in consciousness, such as dissociative identity disorder and dissociative amnesia. Abnormalities in mind-body and perceptual awareness, as in depersonalization/derealization disorder, are common during the acute experience of trauma and may become problems in themselves for some people over long periods of time. Dissociation calls for reintegration, with an emphasis on acknowledging, bearing, and putting into perspective stressors that contribute to the fragmentation of identity, memory, and consciousness. The new dissociative subtype of PTSD highlights the role of dissociation both in regulating strong emotional response to trauma and in suppressing such reactions to the point that treatments that should work, such as prolonged exposure, may instead trigger further dissociation and prevent access to and working-through of trauma-related memories. Recent neuroimaging research has demonstrated that dissociation involves frontal hyperactivity coupled with limbic inhibition, the opposite of what is seen in the hyperarousal types of PTSD. Furthermore, individuals prone to such dissociative responses to trauma are more likely to have a history of early childhood trauma and abuse. Thus, effective treatment involves training in emotion regulation, cognitive restructuring, and danger avoidance, in addition to exposure-based working-through of traumatic memories. Because dissociation is a failure of integration, the treatments for it must integrate emotion, cognition, memory, and somatic control. Even Janet and Freud would likely agree about these fundamental elements, were they able to examine the evidence that has accumulated since their original pioneering writings.

Key Points

- Dissociative disorders often occur in the aftermath of trauma.

- Dissociation buffers stress during trauma but hampers working through it later.

- Dissociation involves frontal hyperactivity and inhibition of limbic activity.

- PTSD typically involves frontal hypoactivity and limbic overactivity.

- DSM-5 includes a new dissociative subtype of PTSD with additional depersonalization/derealization symptoms.

- Dissociative disorders are not rare, with prevalence of about 3% in the general population.

- Treatment of dissociative disorders involves teaching control over dissociative and related affective states.

- Treatments of dissociative and nondissociative types of PTSD differ.

- Phase-oriented treatment with stabilization and reliance on more than exposure is needed for dissociative PTSD.

- Psychotherapy rather than medication is the primary treatment for dissociative disorders.

SUGGESTED READINGS

Brand BL, Lanius R, Vermetten E, et al: Where are we going? An update on assessment, treatment, and neurobiological research in dissociative disorders as we move toward the DSM-5. J Trauma Dissociation 13(1):9–31, 2012 22211439

Cloitre M, Petkova E, Wang J, et al: An examination of the influence of a sequential treatment on the course and impact of dissociation among women with PTSD related to childhood abuse. Depress Anxiety 29(8):709–717, 2012 22550033

Dalenberg CJ, Brand BL, Gleaves DH, et al: Evaluation of the evidence for the trauma and fantasy models of dissociation. Psychol Bull 138(3):550–588, 2012 22409505

Spiegel D, Lewis-Fernández R, Lanius R, et al: Dissociative disorders in DSM-5. Annu Rev Clin Psychol 9:299–326, 2013 23394228

REFERENCES

American Psychiatric Association: Diagnostic and Statistical Manual of Mental Disorders, 4th Edition. Washington, DC, American Psychiatric Association, 1994

American Psychiatric Association: Diagnostic and Statistical Manual of Mental Disorders, 5th Edition. Arlington, VA, American Psychiatric Association, 2013

Breuer J, Freud S: Studies on hysteria (1893–1895), in Standard Edition of the Complete Psychological Works of Sigmund Freud, Vol 2. Translated and edited by Strachey J. London, Hogarth Press, 1955, pp 1–319

Cloitre M, Stovall-McClough KC, Nooner K, et al: Treatment for PTSD related to childhood abuse: a randomized controlled trial. Am J Psychiatry 167(8):915–924, 2010 20595411

Cloitre M, Courtois CA, Charuvastra A, et al: Treatment of complex PTSD: results of the ISTSS expert clinician survey on best practices. J Trauma Stress 24(6):615–627, 2011 22147449

Cloitre M, Petkova E, Wang J, et al: An examination of the influence of a sequential treatment on the course and impact of dissociation among women with PTSD related to childhood abuse. Depress Anxiety 29(8):709–717, 2012 22550033

Dalenberg CJ, Brand BL, Gleaves DH, et al: Evaluation of the evidence for the trauma and fantasy models of dissociation. Psychol Bull 138(3):550–588, 2012 22409505

Daniels JK, Coupland NJ, Hegadoren KM, et al: Neural and behavioral correlates of peritraumatic dissociation in an acutely traumatized sample. J Clin Psychiatry 73(4):420–426, 2012 22394402

Dorahy MJ, Corry M, Shannon M, et al: Complex trauma and intimate relationships: the impact of shame, guilt and dissociation. J Affect Disord 147(1–3):72–79, 2013 23141670

Ebner-Priemer UW, Mauchnik J, Kleindienst N, et al: Emotional learning during dissociative states in borderline personality disorder. J Psychiatry Neurosci 34(3):214–222, 2009 19448852

Etkin A, Wager TD: Functional neuroimaging of anxiety: a meta-analysis of emotional processing in PTSD, social anxiety disorder, and specific phobia. Am J Psychiatry 164(10):1476–1488, 2007 17898336

Felmingham K, Kemp AH, Williams L, et al: Dissociative responses to conscious and non-conscious fear impact underlying brain function in post-traumatic stress disorder. Psychol Med 38(12):1771–1780, 2008 18294420

Foote B, Smolin Y, Kaplan M, et al: Prevalence of dissociative disorders in psychiatric outpatients. Am J Psychiatry 163(4):623–629, 2006 16585436

Francati V, Vermetten E, Bremner JD: Functional neuroimaging studies in posttraumatic stress disorder: review of current methods and findings. Depress Anxiety 24(3):202–218, 2007 16960853

Ginzburg K, Koopman C, Butler LD, et al: Evidence for a dissociative subtype of posttraumatic stress disorder among help-seeking childhood sexual abuse survivors. J Trauma Dissociation 7(2):7–27, 2006 16769663

Hagenaars MA, van Minnen A, Hoogduin KA: The impact of dissociation and depression on the efficacy of prolonged exposure treatment for PTSD. Behav Res Ther 48(1):19–27, 2010 19766987

Hilgard E: Divided Consciousness: Multiple Controls in Human Thought and Action. New York, Wiley-Interscience, 1977

Janet P: L'Automatisme Psychologique. Paris, Felix Alcan, 1889

Jaycox LH, Foa EB, Morral AR: Influence of emotional engagement and habituation on exposure therapy for PTSD. J Consult Clin Psychol 66(1):185–192, 1998 9489273

Kleindienst N, Limberger MF, Ebner-Priemer UW, et al: Dissociation predicts poor response to dialectical behavioral therapy in female patients with borderline personality disorder. J Pers Disord 25(4):432–447, 2011 21838560

Kluft R: Multiple personality disorder, in American Psychiatric Press Annual Review of Psychiatry, Vol 10. Edited by Tasman A, Goldfinger SM. Washington, DC, American Psychiatric Press, 1991, pp 161–188

Lanius RA, Tuhan I: Stage-oriented trauma treatment using dialectical behaviour therapy. Can J Psychiatry 48(2):126–127, 2003 12655913

Lanius RA, Bluhm R, Lanius U, et al: A review of neuroimaging studies in PTSD: heterogeneity of response to symptom provocation. J Psychiatr Res 40(8):709–729, 2006 16214172

Lanius RA, Vermetten E, Loewenstein RJ, et al: Emotion modulation in PTSD: clinical and neurobiological evidence for a dissociative subtype. Am J Psychiatry 167(6):640–647, 2010 20360318

Lanius RA, Brand B, Vermetten E, et al: The dissociative subtype of posttraumatic stress disorder: rationale, clinical and neurobiological evidence, and implications. Depress Anxiety 29(8):701–708, 2012 22431063

Lussier RG, Steiner J, Grey A, et al: Prevalence of dissociative disorders in an acute care day hospital population. Psychiatr Serv 48(2):244–246, 1997 9021860

Paris J: The rise and fall of dissociative identity disorder. J Nerv Ment Dis 200(12):1076–1079, 2012 23197123

Resick PA, Galovski TE, O'Brien Uhlmansiek M, et al: A randomized clinical trial to dismantle components of cognitive processing therapy for posttraumatic stress disorder in female victims of interpersonal violence. J Consult Clin Psychol 76(2):243–258, 2008 18377121

Resick PA, Suvak MK, Johnides BD, et al: The impact of dissociation on PTSD treatment with cognitive processing therapy. Depress Anxiety 29(8):718–730, 2012 22473922

Shin LM, Wright CI, Cannistraro PA, et al: A functional magnetic resonance imaging study of amygdala and medial prefrontal cortex responses to overtly presented fearful faces in posttraumatic stress disorder. Arch Gen Psychiatry 62(3):273–281, 2005 15753240

Spiegel D, Loewenstein RJ, Lewis-Fernández R, et al: Dissociative disorders in DSM-5. Depress Anxiety 28(9):824–852, 2011 21910187

Spiegel D, Lewis-Fernández R, Lanius R, et al: Dissociative disorders in DSM-5. Annu Rev Clin Psychol 9:299–326, 2013 23394228

Stein DJ, Koenen KC, Friedman MJ, et al: Dissociation in posttraumatic stress disorder: evidence from the World Mental Health Surveys. Biol Psychiatry 73(4):302–312, 2013 23059051

Waelde LC, Silvern L, Fairbank JA: A taxometric investigation of dissociation in Vietnam veterans. J Trauma Stress 18(4):359–369, 2005 16281233

Waller NG, Ross CA: The prevalence and biometric structure of pathological dissociation in the general population: taxometric and behavior genetic findings. J Abnorm Psychol 106(4):499–510, 1997 9358680

Weathers FW, Keane TM, Davidson JR: Clinician-Administered PTSD Scale: a review of the first ten years of research. Depress Anxiety 13(3):132–156, 2001 11387733

Wolf EJ, Lunney CA, Miller MW, et al: The dissociative subtype of PTSD: a replication and extension. Depress Anxiety 29(8):679–688, 2012a 22639402

Wolf EJ, Miller MW, Reardon AF, et al: A latent class analysis of dissociation and posttraumatic stress disorder: evidence for a dissociative subtype. Arch Gen Psychiatry 69(7):698–705, 2012b 22752235

CHAPTER 8

Persistent Complex Bereavement Disorder and Its Treatment

M. KATHERINE SHEAR, M.D.
COLLEEN E. GRIBBIN, M.A.

SYNDROME OF COMPLICATED GRIEF

The term *complicated grief* (CG) is used to describe a syndrome consisting of acute grief symptoms that persist beyond the time frame that is considered adaptive or culturally appropriate in the bereaved person's social network accompanied by complicating thoughts, feelings, and behaviors. This syndrome has now been named persistent complex bereavement disorder (PCBD) and is included as a condition for further study in DSM-5 (American Psychiatric Association 2013, pp. 789–792). (There is continuous controversy about the name for this condition; however, in this chapter we use the term PCBD in conjunction with DSM-5 except when referring to research that was published using the term CG.) CG lies at the extreme end of the grief spectrum in terms of severity, and it contains atypical features that derail mourning. The best way to understand grief that follows the death of a loved one is by considering what is known about attachment relationships. Close attachments are biologically motivated, and there are typical ways in which people respond to the loss of someone close. Such a loss creates a destabilized attachment system (acute attachment insecurity) in which the attachment behavioral system is activated while caregiving and exploratory systems are inhibited. The configuration and course of grief differ for each person and each loss. Nevertheless, it is possible to identify generic symptoms of acute grief on the basis of the instinctive response to attachment loss.

TYPICAL ACUTE GRIEF

Typical symptoms of acute grief include separation distress with intense yearning, longing, or searching; preoccupation with thoughts and memories of the lost person that frequently include hallucinatory experiences; pronounced feelings of emotional loneliness; feelings of emptiness and anxiety about a future without that person; feelings of mistrust and detachment from others; and feelings of frustration related to being deprived of someone wanted so desperately. There are often feelings related to a sense of having failed as a caregiver and accompanying self-blaming thoughts. Feelings of guilt or remorse are common, and there is sometimes shame. Loss of a loved one usually inhibits one's motivation to explore the world. In adults this produces feelings of incompetence and disinterest in learning and performing in the world. Additionally, confrontation with death often triggers a trauma response, with feelings of shock and disbelief and a sense of confusion and disorientation.

From a clinical perspective PCBD is a chronic, disabling condition in need of treatment, and clinicians need to know how to recognize its symptoms and to differentiate them from the symptoms of PCBD's nearest neighbors—normal grief, major depression, and posttraumatic stress disorder (PTSD)—because the treatment approach is different for each. Clinicians must make categorical decisions about whether or not to intervene and, if so, how. If clinicians do not understand how to recognize PCBD as different from typical acute grief, they are at risk of intervening in a normal process and perhaps derailing it. At the same time, if clinicians do not detect grief that is prolonged and complicated, and if they fail to see the difference between PCBD and other major depression or PTSD, they may not know how to help, or they may provide ineffective treatment and thereby condemn a bereaved person to continue to suffer symptoms that may respond to treatment.

Although the experience of each person and each loss is unique, there are some discernible commonalities. Clinicians working with grief need to decide whether indicators of progress are present so they can determine whether the process of adaptation is on track. Clinicians need to make categorical decisions. Is the person's grief progressing effectively—yes, no, or maybe? In this chapter we focus on understanding and diagnosing PCBD as the syndrome that results when grief symptoms take over and metastasize, invading the life of the bereaved person.

Acute grief is usually a dynamic response that shifts over time, albeit not in a linear fashion. Adaptation to the loss transforms and integrates the grief through a process that occurs in fits and starts that often seem erratic. With PCBD the course of grief is different. The person with PCBD may be troubled by something related to the loss that cannot be put to rest. There may be troubling circumstances surrounding the death. There may be distressing thoughts that pertain to the deceased. There may be something about the death that creates a seemingly insurmountable problem in the bereaved person's life—a serious threat to his or her physical, social, or psychological well-being. Whatever the issue, one or more stubborn quandaries can thwart the mourning process and stall forward momentum.

The intensity of acute grief, frightening as it is, is a natural part of an adaptive process, but it feels like being lost and disoriented in a storm-tossed sea. Grief surges, threatens to drown the person, and demonstrates no hint of movement toward the shoreline. The person with PCBD continues to have a powerful desire to be with the deceased person on the theory that only this person can restore well-being. For most bereaved people the psychological processes set in motion by the death foster integration—that is, coming to terms with the loss and restoration of meaning and satisfaction to life. For a person with PCBD the processes set in motion by the death foster hopelessness, self-blame, anxiety, resentment, or bitterness and lead to a circular route that remains within the province of acute grief. A patient might say, "I just wasn't progressing" or "Time is moving on but I am not."

There are as yet no official criteria for PCBD, but many studies confirm that PCBD is an important clinical problem. For example, it causes impairment in work and social functioning (Bonanno et al. 2007; Cruz et al. 2007; Melhem et al. 2007; Shear et al. 2006, 2007; Simon et al. 2005, 2007; Zuckoff et al. 2006). Among people with bipolar disorder, the occurrence of CG is associated with more panic disorder, greater suicidality (Simon et al. 2005), and greater sleep disturbance (Maytal et al. 2007). Symptoms of PCBD differ from those of other psychiatric disorders, such as depression or PTSD. Therefore, the DSM-5 Work Group on Anxiety, Obsessive-Compulsive Spectrum, Posttraumatic, and Dissociative Disorders added this condition in the category *other specified trauma- and stressor-related disorder* but did not give it a code number to differentiate it from the other three disorders under this new category in DSM-5 (American Psychiatric Association 2013, p. 289).

PROPOSED PERSISTENT COMPLEX BEREAVEMENT DISORDER CRITERIA

Diagnostic criteria for PCBD were included in Section III of DSM-5 and referenced under the category *other specified trauma- and stressor-related disorders.*

However, data from clinical (C. Mauro, personal communication, 2015) and community (S. Cozza, personal communication, 2015) sources indicate that these criteria are not appropriately sensitive. Therefore, we do not recommend that readers use these criteria.

Diagnostic Features

The essential features of PCBD (see Chapter 3, "Conceptual Framework and Controversies in Adjustment Disorders") include the persistence of characteristic symptoms for more than 12 months (6 months for children) after the death of an important person (Criterion A). PCBD symptoms include intense separation distress and troubling concern(s) about some aspect(s) of the loss (Criterion B). Most people react strongly to the loss of a loved one during the first weeks and months after the death. Bereaved people experience an acute grief response that can be intensely painful and disruptive. The two main differences between this more typical kind of grief and PCBD are 1) that separation distress is exceptionally strong in PCBD and 2) that the bereaved person is bothered a great deal by and focuses much attention on things related to how, when, or why the person died or about the consequences of the death. Most commonly, these symptoms of CG are chronic and persistent and cause clinically significant distress or impairment in functioning (Criterion D) (American Psychiatric Association 2013).

PCBD occurs following loss of a close attachment, someone deeply loved. Although the general view among mental health professionals is that grief is more likely to be problematic if the relationship to the deceased was ambivalent, this is usually not the case. If anything, the opposite is more likely: the most difficult loss is one in which the relationship to the deceased was especially strong and positive and often long lasting. Along these lines, studies suggest that a positive experience with caregiving is associated with greater likelihood of CG (Boerner et al. 2004; Schulz et al. 2006).The stronger the attachment, the more difficult the mourning period will be. But of course, not everyone who had a strong relationship with the deceased person suffers from CG.

Many of the CG patients with whom we have worked are parents who have lost a child in whom they felt a particular pride and from whom they drew special satisfaction, as well as people who have lost a partner whom they considered a soul mate. Loss of a best friend, close confidant, beloved parent, or sibling can also result in CG. One woman with CG—we'll call her Mrs. S—described her deceased spouse in a way that is typical among people with CG:

> He had the prettiest eyes and a very nice smile. He was tall. I wouldn't say he was handsome, but he was handsome to me. He was well built. He was a warm person, very attentive and intelligent. We started going out because he saw me in the

grocery store, and then he saw me there again, and he picked me up. He asked me out. It was nice—a gentleman. He wasn't trying to use me. On our first date, he made me feel good about myself. I was divorced and so was he—he had children, but I got along with them. I went ahead with my life. We had friends together but we each had our own friends too. He was a good cook and he would always cook for me. He would just have me set the table. One thing I didn't like was that he smoked all the time. I didn't approve because I didn't smoke but I put up with it. We shared a lot of interests. The magic part was we could be in the same room and see things that other people didn't see—things about nature or feeling things from people. He didn't have to teach me that. I didn't have to teach him that. There was no trying to change anyone. It was so comfortable. We were soul mates.

A person like Mrs. S who loses someone so close will feel shattered by the loss. When Mrs. S learned of her husband's death, she cried out, "No. No. No. No. It can't be true!" as she slammed her hand on the wall. In the early aftermath of a loss like this, there is commonly a sense of disorientation and confusion as though the simplest task is foreign and impossible to complete. At times, the intense pain alternates with a feeling of being stunned, dazed, numb, and disconnected from feelings altogether. The person may feel that he or she is going through life as an automaton. At other times, numbness is a dominant and persistent feeling, contributing to a sense of disconnection from ongoing life.

Separation distress can be experienced in various ways. Most often there is intense yearning—an overwhelming desire to be with the person again (Criterion B1). The feeling of wanting the person back may be so strong that it is indescribable. The bereaved person may wish that things were the way they were when the loved one was alive or may think that only if the loved one returned could the bereaved person feel OK again. He or she may think about how perfect things were before the loved one died (O'Connor and Sussman 2014). Some people experience an urge to search for the deceased, to do things to find the person who died or to feel connected to him or her. For example, they may spend inordinate amounts of time at the cemetery or keep the cremation ashes close by or "talk" to the person. They may spend time looking at, touching, or smelling the belongings of the deceased. They may spend hours each day looking at pictures or making scrapbooks. In rare cases, the urge to search for the person becomes so strong that the bereaved individual tries to take his or her own life in order to find the deceased loved one (Criteron C7).

The bereaved person may have a recurring sense of disbelief about the death (Criterion C2) or feel unwilling or unable to accept the death (Criterion C1). The person may have difficulty comprehending that the deceased is really gone and not coming back (Criterion C1). He or she may engage in actions that exacerbate this unreality—refusing to empty closets, toss out equipment, or change a telephone listing. The person knows that the loved one has died but does not fully acknowledge it. Some people with PCBD are frequently engrossed in thoughts or images of the deceased (Criterion B3). Occasionally, there may be reveries in which the bereaved person imagines being with the deceased again and may even lose sense of time during these periods of daydreaming. Periods of preoccupation with thoughts or memories of the deceased are common and are seen in many people with PCBD.

In our research studies on CG treatment, we have required participants to have been bereaved for longer than 6 months; most people we have treated in our studies have been bereaved for several years. We suggest that clinicians evaluate people who have experienced bereavement for longer than 6 months but use judgment regarding whether to intervene immediately. If a patient's grief seems to be progressing and the person has good social support, the clinician might want to provide psychoeducation, support, and encouragement for the patient and significant others while monitoring the symptoms for a while.

Distress over circumstances or consequences of the death (Criterion B4) is experienced in several different ways. Many people have thoughts that the death could have been prevented or made easier; they might chastise themselves for not being careful enough (e.g., "If only I had seen it coming, I could have stopped him from dying at this time") or blame others for inattention or neglect (e.g., "I keep thinking about how the medical staff just wrote him off") or think that they cannot manage without this person (e.g., "There is too much to do, and I don't know where to start"). These counterfactual "if only" thoughts or future-oriented catastrophizing thoughts plague the bereaved person and cause considerable distress. The following vignette demonstrates a typical reaction among people with PCBD.

Case Vignette

Mr. H is a 55-year-old man whose 82-year-old mother died. He had been very close to her, yet he was surprised by the intensity of his grief. He sought treatment because he was feeling lost and alone, consumed with thoughts of self-blame and remorse, and spending his days sitting alone in his home. His self-owned business was failing, and his wife was frightened because of this and because he would not communicate with her. Previously, he was happily married and functioned well as an active, community-oriented businessman. Now, no one in his family could reach him emotionally.

Mr. H couldn't stop thinking about sending his mother to hospice care. He said, "I know it was the best thing. They were nice to her, and she was very ill. She didn't have long to live. But then I have this feeling that it was like giving up on her—almost like I didn't care what happened to her—that's what she said, you know. She said, "I am not giving up. I am not ready to die. Don't send me somewhere to die." I keep hearing her say that.

Mr. H said his mother knew how ill she was, or at least the family had told her, but she probably didn't care. He said, "She could be like that—stubborn. She didn't want to know about cancer. She didn't want to hear that this was the end.

And I kind of blame her doctor for this too—he knew her really well and he didn't want to deal with her emotionally, so he offered her experimental treatment. Then he called me and told me that the chances it would work were very low and it could have bad side effects. He told me he did not recommend it...but he didn't tell her that. He left it up to me. It was very frustrating."

Mr. H finally convinced his mother to go into hospice care. He said, "The night she died, she was very weak. I sat with her all through the night. She died at 5 A.M. I was holding her hand. She had lapsed into a kind of coma, around 1 A.M., but the evening before was a nightmare for me. She kept looking at me like I was a murderer and saying, 'Why didn't I get that treatment the doctor recommended? Did you think it was time for me to die? Why didn't he give me that treatment? Maybe it was too expensive. Maybe it's because I am too old. Why didn't you fight for me?' I tried to stay calm and just kept stroking her forehead and telling her I loved her, but inside I was in turmoil."

Recurrent intense feelings of anger or bitterness related to the death (Criterion C4) are common. Bitterness may be directed toward a particular person, such as a family member or friend, a medical professional or member of the clergy, or even the deceased person. Anger or bitterness may also be directed to God or fate.

Excessive avoidance of thoughts, activities, and situations that are reminders of the loss is also common (Criterion C6). People vary in the kinds of things they avoid and may sometimes be unaware of the avoidance. It is helpful for the clinician to ask if there is anything the person used to do when the deceased was alive that he or she is no longer doing. It may also be helpful to ask if there are things the person would do if he or she felt more comfortable. Some people avoid rooms in their own homes, favorite places they went with the deceased, certain activities such as watching movies or listening to music, or even looking at pictures of the deceased. People may have difficulty being at family gatherings or doing things that seem connected to the loved one's death, such as visiting a hospital or funeral home or going to the cemetery. There is often intense psychological or physiological reactivity on exposure to reminders of the person who died.

Emotions are commonly activated at certain difficult times of the year, such as the anniversary of the death, the birthday of the bereaved or the deceased person, other birthdays or wedding anniversaries, and family holidays, including Mother's Day, Father's Day, and the period from Thanksgiving to New Year's Day. A wide range of situations can evoke strong emotions or even physical pain for a person who has lost a close companion because the deceased loved one has shared so many aspects of the person's life. Painful emotions often surge suddenly and unexpectedly, triggered by a thought of the person, by someone else mentioning the name of the deceased or saying something that reminds the person of the deceased, or by a cue in the environment—something as simple as an entrance to a park or eating oatmeal. People sometimes feel that the world is filled with land mines of reminders.

A bereaved person often feels that others do not understand the impact of his or her loss (Criterion C8), and this creates a sense of estrangement and deep loneliness. The person has difficulty engaging fully in ongoing relationships, feeling that he or she can be close only to someone who has experienced a similar loss. Others seem to expect the person to move on and put the pain aside, and this seems impossible to do. Sometimes, there are strong feelings of confusion or uncertainty about one's role in a world without the deceased (Criterion C11) or a feeling that life is empty, meaningless, or unbearable (Criterion C10) because a loved one has died or that joy and satisfaction are no longer possible. There is no light at the end of the tunnel. The person commonly thinks about death. Many people have occasional thoughts that they wish to die and they just need to wait until it happens (Criterion C7). Some wish to take their own lives but are restrained from this by the idea that their loved one would not want this or by religious beliefs. Some people deliberately neglect their health or behave recklessly in order to leave death to chance. Occasionally, suicidal thoughts are strong and persistent and lead to suicide attempts.

Associated Features

Individuals with CG often suffer from sleep disturbance (Germain et al. 2005). They do not usually experience nightmares related to the death, but they might dream about the person who died and feel a wave of grief as they awaken to reminders that the person is gone. Daily life routines (e.g., eating, socializing, exercising) are also frequently disrupted when a loved one dies (Monk et al. 2006), and this can affect the individual's mood and sense of well-being. People with CG often report that they had difficult relationships with caregivers during childhood, and insecure attachment styles, both anxious preoccupied and avoidant, have been found to be associated with elevated rates of CG (Wijngaards-de Meij et al. 2007). Many people with PCBD are highly self-reliant and focused on caregiving in interpersonal relationships. The feeling of vulnerability that accompanies grief is especially difficult for them, which may lead to difficulty accepting support from others. Insecure attachment may interfere with restoring satisfying relationships after an important loss. Feelings of loss of purpose or meaning may dampen enthusiasm for work even when working was previously enjoyable. Survivor guilt or avoidance behavior may create important barriers to restoration of the capacity for joy and satisfaction in social life and leisure activities.

People with CG experience elevated rates of major depression and PTSD and possibly increased rates of other mood and anxiety disorders (Neria et al. 2007; Shear et al. 2006; Silverman et al. 2000). Some studies show an increased rate of separation anxiety disorder with CG, whereas others do not. Somatization and substance use disorders may also be increased with CG.

Associated Laboratory Findings

Findings from some studies suggest that cortisol elevation occurs in CG, and one study shows that activation of the nucleus accumbens on brain imaging differs in women with CG and in a similarly bereaved group without CG (O'Connor et al. 2008). Individuals with CG show deficits in certain biographical and autobiographical memory functions (Boelen et al. 2010; Golden et al. 2007; Maccallum and Bryant 2008, 2010). In particular, findings indicate that bereaved people with CG differ from bereaved people without CG in their ability to generate specific autobiographical memories in response to work cues with positive or negative valence. Those with CG produce more specific memories of the deceased. Additionally, their self-defining memories are more likely to involve the deceased than are those of bereaved individuals without CG. In a study of heart rate response during discussion of a loss, Bonanno et al. (2007) found reduced heart rate among participants with CG and increased heart rate among those with PTSD.

Physical Findings and General Medical Conditions

Little research has been done pertaining to physical illness and PCBD. A few accounts of self-reported symptoms suggest that there may be a risk for new-onset hypertension or the development of neoplastic disease (Chen et al. 1999; Prigerson et al. 1997). Although these reports have not been confirmed, clinicians should be aware of the possibility that PCBD may be a vulnerability factor for physical illness, especially in older adults. Additionally, a person with CG who has indirect suicidal behavior may neglect his or her health, such as by failing to go to needed medical appointments and/or by failing to follow up with treatment or adhere to medication schedules as directed by a physician (Szanto et al. 2006).

Cultural and Age-Related Factors

Culture and age have important roles in acute grief and mourning practices. There is great variation in cultural approaches to mourning, such that in some cultures almost any display of emotion is proscribed and in others prolonged display of mourning is required. Nevertheless, it appears that the syndrome of CG is recognizable across cultures. Studies of CG have been done across cultures within the United States (Cruz et al. 2007; Goldsmith et al. 2008) and among bereaved individuals in western Europe, Iran, Bosnia, Kosovo, Pakistan, Turkey, Rwanda, China, and Japan (Shear et al. 2011).

PCBD occurs in people of all ages. Children endorse similar symptoms as adults, although it is not known whether differences in patterns of symptoms occur across different age groups. For children, the unavailability of a supportive caregiver may be especially important in predisposing them to PCBD. Older adults may have a slightly lower rate of PCBD than younger people.

Prevalence and Course

The prevalence of PCBD is unknown because no epidemiological studies have been done. The best estimate to date is that PCBD occurs in about 7% of bereaved individuals and that certain subgroups may develop PCBD at a higher frequency. For example, it appears that PCBD occurs at higher rates following violent death and that parents who lose children have a longer trajectory of healing. A recent study of parents whose children died in a pediatric intensive care unit showed a 60% rate of CG at 1 year after the death (Meert et al. 2010). A study of suicide survivors found that they had a 20% rate of CG (Mitchell et al. 2004). Other subgroups that may have increased risk for PCBD include people with a history of mood or anxiety disorders, people who have experienced multiple losses, and people who are under exceptional stress at the time of the loss. Individuals who have had difficult relationships with early caregivers may be more prone to develop PCBD.

The issue of parental bereavement deserves special comment. Numerous studies have documented that losing a child leads to the most difficult type of bereavement. There are two views regarding treatment of parental bereavement. One view is that because most parents struggle over a longer period to come to terms with the death of a child, clinicians should not diagnose PCBD in parents using the same time frame as with other bereaved individuals. These parents should be given more time to heal before diagnosis. The other view is that child death is an especially toxic experience and is more likely to trigger PCBD. We offer a medical analogy: If a person is exposed to an especially virulent microorganism, the likelihood that he or she will develop a serious infection is much greater than if the person is exposed to something less toxic; a physician would never refrain from trying to treat someone with an infection just because almost anyone so infected would get sick. If there were no stigma attached to mental health treatment, all people experiencing parental bereavement would probably want the help. We encourage people to participate in CG treatment (CGT) if they are struggling with a very difficult loss, even though we agree that almost anyone would have a hard time with it. In the end, however, this is clearly a decision that patients should and will make for themselves.

Once PCBD is established, its course appears to be chronic and persistent. Symptoms typically develop at the time of the death and can persist for decades if not treated. There have been no long-term studies documenting the proportion of individuals expected to recover without treatment, but the trajectory of improvement appears to be slow. Good social support, including companionship and help with tangible and emotional support, is likely associated with a better prognosis. As grief persists over years and decades, most people find that their support system vanishes. People around someone with PCBD often feel frustrated and helpless, and the person with PCBD knows this. Often, these people become strong allies once they understand the syndrome of PCBD and see their loved one trying to get help. This is one reason CGT includes a session with a significant other. However, when the patient has a serious ongoing conflict with a significant other, this is likely to be associated with a worse outcome.

Differential Diagnosis

At first glance grief seems to resemble depression. But are they really similar? Freud's view that grief and depression are similar has had a big impact on psychiatric thinking. Freud (1917/1974) famously linked mourning and melancholia and hypothesized that depression is the consequence of intrapsychic loss. More recently, clinicians and researchers have struggled with deciding whether depression is a normal consequence of bereavement. Both conditions are associated with symptoms of sad mood, loss of interest in the outside world, loss of energy and concentration, and disturbances in sleep and appetite. Both depression and bereavement commonly incite in the sufferer feelings of guilt and self-blame. However, there are important differences in these symptoms when they occur with grief compared with depression. The preponderance of evidence indicates that not all bereaved people, even those with PCBD, experience depression.

Individuals with PCBD have prominent symptoms that are not seen with depression. They have an intense desire to be with the person who died and may spend hours every day reminiscing and reviewing mementos, or they may enter pleasurable reveries in which they imagine being with the deceased person. For example, Mrs. L sought treatment for PCBD. She arrived at her first treatment session with two shopping bags filled with albums of pictures of her deceased son, Jared. Although tearful, she proudly shared the pictures with her therapist, providing many warm anecdotes and even some funny stories about Jared as she did so. Another patient, Mrs. G, described spending hours every day engrossed in making scrapbooks and crafts from her daughter Sara's possessions. She could temporarily banish her deep sorrow while engaged in these activities. In contrast, depressed patients do not typically feel a passionate connection with someone, and activities do not elevate their mood.

PCBD is associated with intrusion and avoidance symptoms that resemble a trauma-like reaction and that are not typically seen in major depression. Most people with PCBD find that their current life is invaded by thoughts or images of the deceased person that may be either voluntary, as with Mrs. G, or involuntary. Either way, the person with PCBD is often preoccupied with thoughts of the deceased. These thoughts may be focused on reasons why the person did not really need to die or on how life cannot go on without this person. Guilty ruminations typically focus specifically on the relationship with the deceased and usually on certain specific events. This specificity is not typical of depression. People with PCBD are highly emotionally activated when confronted with reminders of the deceased or of the loss. As a consequence, they often seek to avoid these activating reminders. In contrast, neither the activation nor the avoidance is typical of depression, although intrusions and avoidance are seen with PTSD.

PCBD, like PTSD, is triggered by a highly disruptive life event that often elicits a response of confusion, disorientation, and disbelief. Intrusive thoughts, preoccupation, and avoidance behaviors are seen with both, as are sleep disturbance and emotion dysregulation. However, there are also some marked differences between PCBD and PTSD. The inciting event is very different: PTSD follows confrontation with a danger, whereas PCBD follows the loss of a highly valued relationship. Physical danger entails exposure to something destructive that threatens physical harm and affects ongoing feelings of safety as related to this exposure. Physical trauma comprises one or more events that are more or less contained in space and time and that trigger feelings of fear and induce a state of hypervigilance. An adaptive response to trauma entails accurate evaluation of the reality of ongoing threat and relearning a sense of safety. With the exception of situations that entail recurrent exposure (e.g., combat, domestic abuse), actual threat is markedly reduced after the event is over.

CONSIDERATIONS RELATED TO THE ETIOLOGY AND PATHOGENESIS OF PERSISTENT COMPLEX BEREAVEMENT DISORDER

The etiology and pathogenesis of PCBD remain unknown. However, considerable research documents the importance of close relationships in everyday life. Loss of a loved one creates great disruption and requires adaptation. We use Bowlby's (1980) conceptualization of the process of adaptation to loss in which successful adaptation entails 1) acknowledgment of the finality and consequences of the death, 2) a revision of the attachment working model (defined as mental representations for understanding the world, self, and others), and 3) restoration of a sense of purpose and meaning and the possibility for happiness. In the following subsections we describe how the complicating problems of grief work against the achievement of these goals.

Failure to Accept the Death

To move from acute to integrated grief, a person must fully accept the finality of the loss. People with CG are painfully aware that their loved one is gone, but many of the factors described earlier (see "Proposed Persistent Complex Bereavement Disorder Criteria") prevent them from accepting the finality of death. To reverse the process, clinicians must gently urge acceptance by the part of the patient's mind that resists the new reality. The patient must find a way to change the thoughts and feelings that block acceptance; these include negative cognitions such as ideas that the loved one should not have died, that the death could have been prevented, that the death is not fair, that the world should be fair, or that the person left behind can neither function nor ever be happy again without the deceased. For example, if a person believes she cannot function without the deceased, she will not begin to accept the consequences of the death, such as the fact that her husband is no longer bringing home a paycheck or sleeping in her bed or brushing his teeth in the morning.

As all the complicating problems—cognitive, behavioral, emotional, and environmental—are addressed, the notion of accepting the loss no longer seems impossible. Acceptance, in turn, allows for the attachment working model to be revised and life goals to be restored. Both of these occurrences, in turn, foster greater acceptance.

Failure to Revise the Attachment Working Model

When the bereaved refuses to accept the finality of the death, the attachment working model is not revised. Explicit memory gets it; implicit memory lags behind. The unrevised model continues to generate impulses to search and long for the deceased and to seek reunion. These disconcerting sensations of disbelief are likely the felt experience of an unrevised working model. In cases of PCBD, the sense of disbelief is associated with a vague impression or expectation that the deceased person is going to reappear—that the bereaved person will wake up from this nightmare and his or her loved one will be present. In one case, a patient continued to set the table for her husband every night, even though she knew rationally that he would not be there. In setting the table, she could imagine being with him, which blocked the revision of the working model and sustained the yearning, proximity seeking, anxiety, and other negative emotions associated with the separation response.

In time, the sense of disbelief usually retreats. Oscillations between experiencing emotional pain and respite from the pain gradually alter the model, gently coaxing the bereaved toward a full realization of the permanence of his or her loss. Paradoxically, revising the working model allows the bereaved a more, rather than less, satisfying connection to the deceased. In *A Grief Observed*, C. S. Lewis wrote about his wife (whom he referred to as "H."), "And suddenly at the very moment when, so far, I mourned H. least, I remembered her best." (Lewis 1961, p. 44). The sense of deep intuitive connection is paradoxically reestablished when this memory, presumably implicit, has been established. Lewis went on to say, "Indeed it was something (almost) better than memory; an instantaneous, unanswerable impression" (p. 45).

Failure to Redefine Life Goals

A person's adaptation to loss often occurs through oscillations between bouts in which the reality, finality, and pain of the death are acknowledged and moratoria or respites in which the pain is set aside. At the same time, it is important for the person to start to envision a life in which joy and satisfaction are possible. For people with PCBD, the entire process is distorted and bogged down so that there is no forward movement. Rather than gradually coming to terms with the loss, a person with PCBD is either engaged in catastrophizing about its consequences or assiduously avoiding this confrontation. Rather than feeling a sense of respite and the freedom to explore new ideas and behaviors, a person with PCBD engages in avoidance that is restricting and inhibiting. The person does not make use of painful confrontation with the loss for the purpose of growing acceptance; instead, the reality of the death is suffused with further pain associated with the same ideas that block acceptance, or the thoughts of the person take over and distract the person from thinking about the death.

Instead of the oscillations lessening and muting emotion, the painful or intrusive thoughts increase in magnitude, and rather than serving the purpose of processing the loss, engagement takes the form of rumination or reveries. Rather than naturally and comfortably setting aside thoughts of the deceased, bereaved individuals may organize their lives to avoid reminders. In essence, the natural oscillation of bouts and moratoria is not productive. There is an absence of a sense of movement. Correspondingly, rather than a respite or breathing space, used to refuel the difficult process of acceptance, turning away from thoughts that trigger emotional pain is the sole, desperate manner of controlling these thoughts.

COMPLICATED GRIEF TREATMENT

CGT is a 16-session efficacy-tested approach (K. Shear et al. 2005, M. K. Shear et al. 2004; M.K. Shear, C. F. Reynolds, and N. S Simon, et al., "Optimizing treatment of complicated grief: a multicenter randomized clinical trial," submitted manuscript, 2015) that contains seven core content modules: psychoeducation, self-regulation, rebuilding connection, aspirational goals, revisiting the story of the death, revisiting the world, and memories past and future. The treatment is usually administered in four phases: getting started, core revisiting sequence, midcourse review, and closing sequence. Throughout the treatment the therapist encourages oscillation between confronting pain and setting it aside, mirroring the process described by Bowlby (1980). Each session entails some work on loss (past focus) and some on restoration (future focus), following the idea put forward by Stroebe and Schut (1999) that loss and restoration are best addressed in tandem. Throughout the treatment, the therapist works to facilitate the three

main processes described by Bowlby: acknowledging the death and its consequences, revising the mental representation of the deceased, and redefining life
goals and plans (see Chapter 9, "Therapeutic Adaptations of Resilience").

CGT has been studied in three National Institute of Mental Health–funded
prospective randomized controlled trials, two of which compared it with standard grief-focused interpersonal psychotherapy (IPT; Shear et al. 2005, 2014)
and one which compared it with pill placebo and CG-informed clinical management (Shear et al., in preparation). In each of these studies, CGT showed significantly better response than did the IPT control. Participants in these studies
have been diverse with respect to age, race, relationship to the deceased, and circumstances of death. Although not definitive, the results to date have not revealed moderation of outcome based on any of these variables.

The introductory sessions (getting started) focus on gathering information
and introducing the treatment. Grief is assessed by both clinical interview and the
administration of rating scales, some of which are used throughout the treatment
in a form of measurement-based care. These include the Inventory of Complicated
Grief (Prigerson et al. 1995), Grief-Related Avoidance Questionnaire (Shear et al.
2007), Typical Beliefs Questionnaire (Skritskaya et al., in preparation), and Work
and Social Adjustment Scale (Mundt et al. 2002). Psychoeducation focuses on our
model of CG as well as an overview of the rationale and procedures to be used. We
present the idea that grief is a form of love and is not pathological and state that a
successful outcome of treatment would be that grief can find its rightful place in
the patient's life. Thoughts and memories of the deceased loved one usually remain
accessible and bittersweet, and there is a continued feeling of connection to the
person who died in a way that honors love and their life together.

In session 1 the therapist introduces a grief monitoring diary, which the patient continues to use throughout treatment. This is a simple tool that asks the
patient to rate grief intensity each day on a scale from 1 to 10. The patient rates
the highest, lowest, and average levels for the day and makes a brief note about
what was happening at each time (Turret and Shear 2012). In session 2 the therapist introduces a focus on aspirational life goals, which is continued during the
last 10 minutes of each session for the remainder of the treatment and is included as a between-session assignment each week. Session 3 is generally held
with a significant other to explain the CGT model and outline the treatment
procedures. The patient and his or her significant other are invited to consider
how the significant other might be helpful in some aspect of the program. Sessions 4–9 focus on the imaginal revisiting procedure, in which patients are
asked to close their eyes and visualize themselves at the time when they first
learned of the death and to tell the story of what happened from that point forward. This procedure is similar to prolonged exposure for PTSD.

Situational revisiting focuses on daily life activities that the patient is avoiding.
Confronting these situations is useful in fostering acknowledgment of the death

and emotion processing and in removing restrictions on the person's ongoing life. During both imaginal and situational revisiting, the patient is asked to report levels of distress in subjective units of distress, rated on a scale from 0 to 100. The final two procedures include some structured memories work and an imaginal conversation with the deceased. These procedures are designed to reinforce a deep sense of connection to the person who died. The patient is also invited to bring in pictures of the deceased. Following successful completion of the revisiting exercises, patients are encouraged to have an imaginal conversation in which they talk with the deceased loved one and then take the loved one's role and answer for him or her. The therapist facilitates this "two-way" conversation as needed. The final component of the treatment is work on treatment termination. Feelings about ending the treatment are reviewed along with treatment gains and plans for the future.

THEORETICAL UNDERPINNINGS OF COMPLICATED GRIEF TREATMENT

In CGT, CG is considered to be a consequence of the disruption of a strong affectional bond. Attachment theory and its accompanying research findings explain the critical role that close relationships play in human lives. The motivation to seek, form, maintain, and respond to the loss of these relationships is considered to be inborn. Meaningful separation from a secure attachment provokes a state of acute attachment insecurity, most prominently described as separation distress with symptoms of attachment activation entailing cognitive, behavioral, and emotional proximity seeking. These are the symptoms of acute grief. Bowlby (1988) viewed the optimal functioning of the attachment behavioral system as important for the maintenance of emotional stability and mental health, sense of self, and positive attitudes toward others. A well-functioning attachment system supports other important biobehavioral functions such as exploration (the motivation to engage the world to work, play, discover, and create) and caregiving (the motivation to provide a secure base and safe haven for a relationship partner).

Researchers have begun to identify brain circuitry that might be involved in the attachment system (e.g., through functional magnetic resonance imaging studies) (Bartels and Zeki 2004). However, according to Coan (2010), another neurobiological attachment researcher, the entire brain is a social brain. To date, there is no agreement about specific circuitry underlying attachment functioning. Nevertheless, in CGT we make the assumption that implicit and explicit memory; positive and negative emotion centers; and cognitive centers for self-monitoring, attention, appraisal, goal-setting, and planning are linked in a functional way in the attachment working model and enable effective functioning of attachment relationships.

Secure attachments are rewarding, provide a foundation of support and shared competence, and play an important role in regulating the partners' emotional and physiological functioning. Bereavement creates a state of acute attachment insecurity. Adaptation to loss requires resolution of this acute attachment insecurity, which in turn relies on assimilation of information about the finality and consequences of the loss. People with CG do not accomplish this resolution because of their inability to assimilate this information into the working model.

It is natural to resist accepting the finality of death, and this resistance leads to ambivalence about admitting the reality of a death. Nevertheless, most people gradually incorporate knowledge of the death into the internal representation of the deceased, and the working model is correspondingly amended in a way that modifies expectations of the deceased loved one and facilitates the potential for restoration of activities and relationships. CGT has two main aims: 1) to resolve grief complications and 2) to foster and reinvigorate the interrupted instinctive process of adapting to the loss. The treatment utilizes a gently structured approach with seven core procedural modules. The treatment draws on Bowlby's (1980) idea that oscillation between confronting emotional pain and avoiding it ("defensive exclusion") is a natural process during bereavement and one that facilitates a gradual process of adaptation. This oscillation toward and away from emotional pain is one of several emotion regulation strategies used in CGT.

CGT is informed by several other theories. One is the dual process model of coping with bereavement, in which Stroebe and Schut (1999) organize bereavement coping as either loss oriented, referring to processing grief and attending to what has been lost, or restoration oriented, referring to coping with the stressors entailed in living without the deceased loved one. CGT incorporates the dual process model idea that a bereaved person needs to address both loss- and restoration-related issues in each of the 16 treatment sessions.

Three other theoretical models are used in CGT: self-determination theory (Deci and Ryan 2000), self-compassion theory (Gilbert 2009; Neff 2011), and the theory of synthetic happiness or the adaptive unconscious (Gilbert et al. 1998). Deci and Ryan (2000) claim that there are basic human needs for autonomy, competence, and relatedness that operate across different age, gender, and cultural groups. There is now considerable evidence supporting this idea. CGT posits that loss of an attachment figure disrupts the ability to meet these needs and that one of the important components of adaptation is to reactivate these goals. Through CGT, we work to help patients find new ways to express intrinsic, autonomous interests and values; to feel competent; and to reestablish meaningful relationships.

CGT also uses self-compassion theory (Gilbert 2009; Neff 2011). Clinicians help patients with CG to treat themselves with kindness rather than criticize themselves for their continued suffering. Patients are encouraged to consider that suffering and acting imperfectly are important universalities of human life. Clinicians further coach patients to practice mindfulness when confronting painful emotions—that is, to work to keep these feelings in perspective. Additionally, CGT is based on a premise that adaptation to loss is a natural process that operates out of awareness, in the implicit system. According to Gilbert and Wilson (2000), this process is especially strongly activated when individuals face a threat to their psychological well-being that is severe and out of their control.

CONTROVERSIES ABOUT PERSISTENT COMPLEX BEREAVEMENT DISORDER

It is common to have controversies with a newly proposed diagnosis for any taxonomy, and DSM-5 is no exception. We have tried to underscore the difference between the cohort who need treatment and individuals experiencing normal bereavement, which is ubiquitous. Important controversies related to the diagnosis of PCBD are summarized below.

- Should there be a time frame for diagnosis of PCBD, and if so, what should it be?
- What criteria are best to ensure identification of people who have PCBD without including bereaved people who do not have it? Can PCBD be clearly differentiated from normal grief?
- Can PCBD be clearly distinguished from depression?
- Should diagnostic criteria be different depending on the way the person died; for example, is violent death different from expected death from illness?
- Should diagnostic criteria be different depending on who died; for example, is the death of child different from the death of an adult?
- Are there important differences in PCBD in children compared with adults?
- Do grief and/or PCBD manifest differently in different cultures?

It is the intent of this chapter to bring a new approach to the understanding of PCBD so that select persons may be offered treatment to manage their troubled mental state

---

Key Points

- Persistent complex bereavement disorder (PCBD) is a syndrome consisting of acute grief symptoms that persist beyond the time frame that is considered adaptive or culturally appropriate, accompanied by complicating thoughts, feelings, and behaviors.

- Complicating problems—cognitive, behavioral, emotional, and environmental—interfere with the natural adaptive response to a loss and result in failure to accept the death and to redefine life goals.

- PCBD affects an estimated 7% of bereaved people and can follow the loss of any close relationship; however, it is more prevalent after the loss of a child or partner and after a sudden or violent death.

- Characteristic symptoms include intense yearning and longing, preoccupation with thoughts of the deceased, a sense of disbelief about or difficulty accepting the loss, emotional distress related to the circumstances or consequences of the loss, and excessive avoidance of reminders.

- PCBD is a chronic, disabling condition in need of treatment, and it is important for clinicians to know how to recognize its symptoms and to differentiate them from typical grief, major depressive disorder, and posttraumatic stress disorder.

- Randomized controlled trials provide support for the efficacy of complicated grief treatment (CGT), which is a 16-session targeted psychotherapy that aims to resolve grief complications and to invigorate the natural adaptive response to a loss.

- CGT is a gently structured treatment that incorporates both loss (past focus) and restoration (future focus) procedures in each of the 16 treatment sessions and contains seven core content modules: psychoeducation, self-regulation, rebuilding connection, aspirational goals, revisiting the story of the death, revisiting the world, and memories past and future.

SUGGESTED READINGS AND WEB SITE

Readings

Neimeyer RA (ed): Techniques of Grief Therapy: Creative Practices for Counseling the Bereaved. New York, Routledge, 2012

Shear MK: Getting straight about grief. Depress Anxiety 29:461–464, 2012

Shear MK: Complicated grief. N Engl J Med 372(2):153–160, 2015

Web Site

Center for Complicated Grief: www.complicatedgrief.org

REFERENCES

American Psychiatric Association: Diagnostic and Statistical Manual of Mental Disorders, 5th Edition, Arlington, VA, American Psychiatric Association, 2013

Bartels A, Zeki S: The neural correlates of maternal and romantic love. Neuroimage 21(3):1155–1166, 2004 15006682

Boelen PA, Huntjens RJ, van Deursen DS, et al: Autobiographical memory specificity and symptoms of complicated grief, depression, and posttraumatic stress disorder following loss. J Behav Ther Exp Psychiatry 41(4):331–337, 2010 20394916

Boerner K, Schulz R, Horowitz A: Positive aspects of caregiving and adaptation to bereavement. Psychol Aging 19(4):668–675, 2004 15584791

Bonanno GA, Neria Y, Mancini A, et al: Is there more to complicated grief than depression and posttraumatic stress disorder? A test of incremental validity. J Abnorm Psychol 116(2):342–351, 2007 17516766

Bowlby J: Loss and Attachment, Vol 3. New York, Basic Books, 1980

Bowlby J: A Secure Base: Parent-Child Attachment and Healthy Human Development. New York, Basic Books, 1988

Chen JH, Bierhals AJ, Prigerson HG, et al: Gender differences in the effects of bereavement-related psychological distress in health outcomes. Psychol Med 29(2):367–380, 1999 10218927

Coan JA: Adult attachment and the brain. J Soc Pers Relat 27(2):210–217, 2010

Cruz M, Scott J, Houck P, et al: Clinical presentation and treatment outcome of African Americans with complicated grief. Psychiatr Serv 58(5):700–702, 2007 17463353

Deci EL, Ryan RM: The "what" and "why" of goal pursuits: human needs and the self-determination of behavior. Psychol Inq 11:227–268, 2000

Freud S: Mourning and melancholia, in The Standard Edition of the Complete Psychological Works of Sigmund Freud, Vol 14. Translated and edited by Strachey J. London, Hogarth Press, 1917/1974, pp 1057–1961

Germain A, Caroff K, Buysse DJ, et al: Sleep quality in complicated grief. J Trauma Stress 18(4):343–346, 2005 16281231

Gilbert DT, Wilson TD: Miswanting: some problems in the forecasting of future affective states, in Feeling and Thinking: The Role of Affect in Social Cognition. Edited by Forgas J. New York, Cambridge University Press, 2000, pp 178–197

Gilbert DT, Pinel EC, Wilson TD, et al: Immune neglect: a source of durability bias in affective forecasting. J Pers Soc Psychol 75(3):617–638, 19998 9781405

Gilbert P: The Compassionate Mind: A New Approach to Life's Challenges. London, Constable and Robinson, 2009

Golden AM, Dalgleish T, Mackintosh B: Levels of specificity of autobiographical memories and of biographical memories of the deceased in bereaved individuals with and without complicated grief. J Abnorm Psychol 116(4):786–795, 2007 18020724

Goldsmith B, Morrison RS, Vanderwerker LC, et al: Elevated rates of prolonged grief disorder in African Americans. Death Stud 32(4):352–365, 2008 18850684

Lewis CS: A Grief Observed. New York, HarperCollins, 1961

Maccallum F, Bryant RA: Self-defining memories in complicated grief. Behav Res Ther 46(12):1311–1315, 2008 18977471

Maccallum F, Bryant RA: Impaired autobiographical memory in complicated grief. Behav Res Ther 48(4):328–334, 2010 20100607

Maytal G, Zalta AK, Thompson E, et al: Complicated grief and impaired sleep in patients with bipolar disorder. Bipolar Disord 9(8):913–917, 2007 18076543

Meert KL, Donaldson AE, Newth CJ, et al: Eunice Kennedy Shriver National Institute of Child Health and Human Development Collaborative Pediatric Critical Care Research Network: Complicated grief and associated risk factors among parents following a child's death in the pediatric intensive care unit. Arch Pediatr Adolesc Med 164(11):1045–1051, 2010 21041597

Melhem NM, Moritz G, Walker M, et al: Phenomenology and correlates of complicated grief in children and adolescents. J Am Acad Child Adolesc Psychiatry 46(4):493–499, 2007 17420684

Mitchell AM, Kim Y, Prigerson HG, et al: Complicated grief in survivors of suicide. Crisis 25(1):12–18, 2004 15384652

Monk TH, Houck PR, Shear MK: The daily life of complicated grief patients—what gets missed, what gets added? Death Stud 30(1):77–85, 2006 16296562

Mundt JC, Marks IM, Shear MK, Greist JH: The Work and Social Adjustment Scale: a simple measure of impairment in functioning. Br J Psychiatry 180(5):461–464, 2002 11983645

Neff KD: Self-Compassion: The Proven Power of Being Kind to Yourself. New York, William Morrow, 2011

Neria Y, Gross R, Litz B, et al: Prevalence and psychological correlates of complicated grief among bereaved adults 2.5–3.5 years after September 11th attacks. J Trauma Stress 20(3):251–262, 2007 17597124

O'Connor MF, Sussman TJ: Developing the Yearning in Situations of Loss Scale: convergent and discriminant validity for bereavement, romantic breakup, and homesickness. Death Stud 38(6–10):450–458, 2014 24758215

O'Connor MF, Wellisch DK, Stanton AL, et al: Craving love? Enduring grief activates brain's reward center. Neuroimage 42(2):969–972, 2008 18559294

Prigerson HG, Maciejewski PK, Reynolds CF 3rd, et al: Inventory of Complicated Grief: a scale to measure maladaptive symptoms of loss. Psychiatry Res 59(1–2):65–79, 1995 8771222

Prigerson HG, Bierhals AJ, Kasl SV, et al: Traumatic grief as a risk factor for mental and physical morbidity. Am J Psychiatry 154(5):616–623, 1997 9137115

Prigerson HG, Horowitz MJ, Jacobs SC, et al: Prolonged grief disorder: psychometric validation of criteria proposed for DSM-V and ICD-11. PLoS Med 6(8):e1000121, 2009 19652695

Schulz R, Boerner K, Shear K, et al: Predictors of complicated grief among dementia caregivers: a prospective study of bereavement. Am J Geriatr Psychiatry 14(8):650–658, 2006 16861369

Shear K, Frank E, Houck PR, Reynolds CF 3rd: Treatment of complicated grief: a randomized controlled trial. JAMA 293(21):2601–2608, 2005 15928281

Shear KM, Jackson CT, Essock SM, et al: Screening for complicated grief among Project Liberty service recipients 18 months after September 11, 2001. Psychiatr Serv 57(9):1291–1297, 2006 16968758

Shear K, Monk T, Houck P, et al: An attachment-based model of complicated grief including the role of avoidance. Eur Arch Psychiatry Clin Neurosci 257(8):453–461, 2007 17629727

Shear MK, Simoon N, Wall M, et al: Complicated grief and related bereavement issues for DSM-5. JAMA Depress Anxiety 28(2):103–117, 2011 21284063

Shear MK, Wang Y, Skritskaya N, et al: Treatment of complicated grief in elderly persons: a randomized clinical trial. JAMA Psychiatry 71(11):1287–1295, 2014 25250737

Silverman GK, Jacobs SC, Kasl SV, et al: Quality of life impairments associated with diagnostic criteria for traumatic grief. Psychol Med 30(4):857–862, 2000 11037094

Simon NM, Pollack MH, Fischmann D, et al: Complicated grief and its correlates in patients with bipolar disorder. J Clin Psychiatry 66(9):1105–1110, 2005 16187766

Simon NM, Shear KM, Thompson EH, et al: The prevalence and correlates of psychiatric comorbidity in individuals with complicated grief. Compr Psychiatry 48(5):395–399, 2007 17707245

Stroebe M, Schut H: The dual process model of coping with bereavement: rationale and description. Death Stud 23(3):197–224, 1999 10848151

Szanto K, Shear MK, Houck PR, et al: Indirect self-destructive behavior and overt suicidality in patients with complicated grief. J Clin Psychiatry 67(2):233–239, 2006 16566618

Turret N, Shear MK: Grief monitoring diary, in Techniques of Grief Therapy: Creative Practices for Counseling the Bereaved. Edited by Neimeyer RA. New York, Routledge, 2012, pp 27–29

Wijngaards-de Meij L, Stroebe M, Schut H, et al: Patterns of attachment and parents' adjustment to the death of their child. Pers Soc Psychol Bull 33(4):537–548, 2007 17363759

Zuckoff A, Shear K, Frank E, et al: Treating complicated grief and substance use disorders: a pilot study. J Subst Abuse Treat 30(3):205–211, 2006 16616164

CHAPTER 9

Therapeutic Adaptations of Resilience

HELPING PATIENTS OVERCOME THE EFFECTS OF TRAUMA AND STRESS

Brian M. Iacoviello, Ph.D.
Dennis S. Charney, M.D.

VARIED REACTIONS TO TRAUMA AND STRESS

Mental health practitioners, as well as emergency room or primary care physicians, are likely to encounter patients who have recently experienced trauma or significant stressors. The kinds of challenges these patients face include abuse or neglect; natural or manmade disasters; significant occupational, family, economic, or other stressors; and subsequent adjustment, mood, anxiety, or substance use disorders. In fact, there is a range of potential responses to stress and trauma. On the one hand, research studies have demonstrated strong associations between the presence of psychiatric disorders and a history of trauma exposure, with the most severe and impairing manifestations being posttraumatic stress disorder (PTSD), depressive disorders, and substance use disorders. On the other hand, it is noteworthy that in most cases, trauma exposure does not lead to psychiatric disorders. For example, one high-quality study based on a

155

large community sample found that the risk of developing PTSD after a traumatic event was approximately 9% (Breslau et al. 1998). However, the prevalence of subsyndromal or other sequelae, such as adjustment disorders or interpersonal or occupational impairment after trauma exposure, is likely much greater. Still, some individuals exhibit a remarkable ability to endure and recover from unfathomable stress, torture, trauma, and disaster. *Resilience,* as a psychosocial construct, is generally described as the adaptive characteristics of an individual to cope with and recover from (and sometimes even thrive after) adversity.

Considering the range of stressful and traumatic experiences that humans can face and the range of potential responses, the factors that contribute to resilience are important to understand. Understanding these factors can help promote resilience and can inform psychosocial intervention strategies for treating trauma survivors.

Anecdotal evidence from interviews with resilient individuals and empirical evidence from research studies of trauma and disaster survivors suggest that a constellation of psychosocial factors contributes to resilience after trauma exposure. The literature has also identified neurobiological factors that appear to influence resilience, including genetic factors, neurochemical systems involved in the stress response, and the functioning of specific neural networks (Feder et al. 2009), although these factors are beyond the scope of this chapter. Our goal in this chapter is to discuss some of the psychosocial factors that have been shown to contribute to resilience, techniques to assess for their presence and identify opportunities for intervention, ways to offer immediate intervention to address these factors and promote resilience, and implications for intervention to enhance resilience after trauma exposure when psychiatric symptoms are present or emerging.

WHAT TO LOOK FOR: THE PSYCHOSOCIAL FACTORS ASSOCIATED WITH RESILIENCE

When a clinician encounters a patient who has experienced trauma or significant stress, assessment of the psychosocial factors associated with resilience is an integral first step to intervention. This assessment is ideally done in collaboration with the patient, as a nonjudgmental discussion to gather information and identify ways to help him or her. A standardized self-report assessment tool, such as the Connor-Davidson Resilience Scale (CD-RISC; Connor and Davidson 2003), may be used to help the clinician identify 1) areas of strength and relative weakness regarding the psychosocial factors associated with resilience and 2) opportunities for intervention. In the following subsections, we describe the factors to assess and suggest ways to probe for their presence. This information is summarized in Table 9–1.

TABLE 9–1.   Components of psychosocial factors promoting resilience in individuals

Factor	Components
Optimism	Maintaining positive expectancies for the future
Cognitive flexibility	Reappraising, reframing, and assimilating traumatic experiences Accepting stress (trauma) and failure as ingredients for growth
Physical health	Engaging in physical activity and exercise
Active coping skills	Actively seeking help and resources Minimizing continued appraisal of threat Maintaining positive self-regard
Social support network	Maintaining a social support network Feeling connected and not isolated
Personal moral compass	Maintaining a sense of purpose in life Engaging in altruistic behavior Maintaining faith/spirituality

Optimism

Optimism refers to the maintenance of positive expectancies for important future outcomes (Carver et al. 2010). Optimism has generally been considered to be a personality dimension, suggesting that it is more like a trait than a state characteristic; however, an individual's degree of optimism can shift over time or across situations. In research studies optimism has been associated with psychosocial well-being among long-term cancer survivors, with psychological adjustment during a life transition, and with lower posttraumatic symptom levels after disasters. Maintaining optimism for the future can buoy one's spirit and provide the stamina to endure stress or trauma. However, optimism alone is not sufficient to foster resilience. The following is the response of James Stockdale, a naval officer held as a prisoner of war in Vietnam and known for his resilience to this situation, to the question "Who did not make it out of Vietnam?"

> Oh, that's easy, the optimists. Oh, they were the ones who said, "We're going to be out by Christmas." And Christmas would come, and Christmas would go. Then they'd say, "We're going to be out by Easter." And Easter would come, and Easter would go. And then Thanksgiving, and then it would be Christmas again. And they died of a broken heart. (Collins 2014)

Cognitive Flexibility

Stockdale's response illuminates another important factor for resilience: *cognitive flexibility*, which refers to the ability to reappraise one's perception and experience of a traumatic situation instead of being rigid. Reappraisal can also involve finding meaning and positive outcomes as well as acknowledging the negative and painful consequences. Cognitive flexibility enables one to reevaluate a traumatic experience and alter the perceived value and meaningfulness of the event. If one can learn to reframe one's thoughts about a traumatic event and assimilate these thoughts into one's memories and beliefs about the event, one may be able to accept and eventually recover. Acceptance and assimilation of a traumatic experience into one's life narrative involve acknowledging that experiences with stress, or even trauma, can provide opportunities for growth. Together, optimism and cognitive flexibility allow an individual to maintain faith that he or she will prevail or survive regardless of the difficulties at hand and, at the same time, confront and accept the brutal facts of his or her current reality.

Active Coping Skills and Social Support Network

Resilient individuals tend to use active rather than passive coping skills; they act and create their own resilience. These skills include being mindful of one's thoughts about the situations in which one finds oneself and actively minimizing the appraisal of threat (but not denying threat) so as not to become consumed by fear, attempting to create positive statements about oneself and one's situation, and making active efforts to seek the help and support of others. These skills are also associated with another important factor for promoting resilience: establishing and nurturing a social support network. Very few people can "go it alone," and resilient individuals often acknowledge the invaluable role of their social support network, which can include the clinician. Considerable emotional strength accrues from close relationships with people and even organizations. Also, the perception of an available "safety net" can enable one to act in one's own interest when confronting or recovering from stressful or traumatic situations. Recent studies of PTSD in veterans returning from wars in Iraq and Afghanistan support this statement. In one study, PTSD symptom severity was associated with greater difficulties in relationships, less social support, and poorer social functioning. Importantly, this was not just a consequence of PTSD; reduced social support and availability of secure relationships mediated the association between PTSD and poor social functioning (Tsai et al. 2012), suggesting that these are important contributors to resilient outcomes. Moreover, some research has suggested that having social supports in place can influence one's thinking about oneself and one's world in a positive way, protecting against hopelessness (Panzarella et al. 2006). Taken together, not feeling alone can engender strength to face fear and trauma, and having effective social support can minimize the experience of hopelessness while encouraging adaptive and active coping. These factors increase the likelihood of resilient outcomes versus psychopathology.

Physical Health

Physical activity is a factor that is primarily behavioral in nature. Attending to one's own physical well-being before, during, and after stress or trauma can promote resilience. Physical exercise improves physical hardiness, which in and of itself can increase the chances of survival from certain traumatic situations. Along with the positive effects that physical exercise confers on mood and self-esteem (Scully et al. 1998), being mindful of one's physical hardiness during a traumatic situation can contribute to mental fortitude to endure and survive. Improved mood and increased self-esteem after experiencing a traumatic situation could also make establishing and nurturing social and interpersonal relationships easier, which, as noted in the previous subsection, is an important factor in promoting resilience.

Personal Moral Compass

A personal moral compass involves developing and holding a set of core beliefs that are positive about oneself and one's role in the world and strong enough that few things can shatter them. Contributing to these core beliefs is the perception that one has of one's own behaviors. Engaging in positive or altruistic behavior toward others can result in positive core beliefs; therefore, altruism is an important behavioral component of developing and embracing a personal moral compass, and, in fact, altruism has been strongly associated with resilience in children and adults (Leontopoulou 2010; Southwick et al. 2005). Altruistic behavior, or other behavior that confers a sense of community and connectedness, can also contribute to perceived meaning and purpose in life, which are also components of embracing a personal moral compass. In several studies, a sense of one's purpose in life has emerged as a key factor associated with resilience and recovery (Alim et al. 2008).

For many people, faith in conjunction with religion or spirituality is also an important component of a personal moral compass. Religion and spirituality can provide opportunities for people to ask questions about and gain some understanding about life and personal meaning when facing traumatic situations. This faith and understanding can aid in constructing personal narratives involving healthy perspectives of traumatic situations and, accordingly, contribute to resilience in the face of trauma. Many studies have investigated the relationship between religious involvement and mental health. Positive religious coping has been associated with better physical and mental outcomes in response to a range of situations, from disasters (e.g., large-scale floods; Smith et al. 2000) to medical illnesses (Pargament et al. 2004).

WHAT TO DO: ENCOURAGING AND ENHANCING PSYCHOSOCIAL FACTORS THAT PROMOTE RESILIENCE

After assessing a patient in relation to the factors described in the previous section, the clinician will be able to identify some that can be addressed or enhanced to promote resilience. Intervening at this point involves taking a clear and direct approach with the patient regarding the opportunities the clinician identifies for growth and resilience and not focusing on "what is wrong." A positive, "you-can-do-it" attitude, coupled with encouragement from the clinician that "these techniques have helped others and can help you," can go a long way in cultivating optimism, gaining the patient's trust in the recommendations, building a therapeutic alliance, and motivating him or her to do the difficult work ahead. Last, the clinician should be prepared to take a hands-on approach. Because a supportive social network is integral to promoting resilience, the clinician should be prepared to become a part of this network over the short term to ensure that the patient embraces and follows the recommendations. This could mean checking in with the patient some time after the original encounter to follow up on the recommendations made, gauge progress, encourage continued effort, or tweak the recommendations on the basis of feedback from the patient after attempting to follow the recommendations. For situations in which a clinician chooses to provide more intervention (e.g., psychotherapy), we also provide recommendations for therapy approaches that are particularly relevant for trauma and promoting resilience when psychiatric symptoms are present or emerging (see later section "Implications for Psychosocial Interventions to Promote Resilience After Trauma").

Encourage Optimism and Attend to Pessimism

Overtly optimistic attitudes can be hard for a patient to cultivate during times of stress or trauma, and often the most a clinician can do in this regard is to hold some of that optimism in view of the patient. This can include expressing hope that the patient's symptoms can improve and citing research and personal experience that certain things like the recommendations the clinician is making have helped others. A positive attitude expressed by the clinician can go a long way in encouraging some hope in the patient, gaining the patient's trust in those recommendations, and motivating him or her to continue to try. Unlike optimistic attitudes, negative or hopeless attitudes seem easy to develop during times of distress. Clinicians should look for and address particularly negative or hopeless attitudes when encountered. They also should attend to common cognitive distortions (Burns 1989) that underlie anxious and depressed thinking, such as all-or-nothing thinking, overgeneralizing, disqualifying the positive, jumping to conclusions, catastrophizing, excessive "should" statements, and personalizing. Studies have also shown that hopelessness in particular can often stem from maintaining rigid and extreme negative core beliefs regarding the stability (enduring over time), globality (permeating different areas of one's life), and internality (regarding the role of one's own personal characteristics) of the negative life events encountered (Alloy et al. 1997). Conversely, maintaining relatively positive core beliefs results in more adaptive thinking in the face of negative life events, which helps in preventing the development of hopelessness and encourages resilience. When clinicians encounter these cognitive distortions or negative beliefs, they could point out the "common thinking trap" to the patient and suggest less biased or negative alternatives to challenge and reframe thoughts about and to encourage a more optimistic attitude toward the future.

Find and Identify With a Resilient Role Model

Role models can often be found in one's own life. A resilient role model is someone who has overcome adversity, disaster, or trauma. Imitation or modeling can be a powerful mode of learning throughout the life span, and finding a resilient role model can be an effective way of cultivating resilience-promoting characteristics via modeling and internalizing the experience of resilience. For example, a role model who has experienced and successfully navigated a traumatic life event can model cognitive flexibility, particularly the experience of acceptance, reappraisal, and assimilation of traumatic experiences. That person can become an integral part of a patient's supportive social network, model active coping skills, and encourage adaptive behavior. He or she can also model the search for purpose in life and provide spiritual awareness and guidance. Clinicians should help direct patients to potential resilient role models. A clinician can ask a patient whether he or she knows anyone who has encountered a similar situation or another traumatic situation and was able to cope and whether the patient thinks this is someone to whom the patient could reach out for advice about how to handle his or her own situation. Resilient role models may also be identified in support groups or other groups for individuals who have encountered similar kinds of stress or trauma.

Establish a Supportive Social Network

As noted earlier, few people can go it alone. Having a social support network to learn from before traumatic experiences and to rely on during and after trauma exposure can be a valuable resource and can mean the difference between resilient outcomes on the one hand and the development of severe psychopathology on the other. Close relations with others can contribute to emotional strength. Social support can influence one's perception of oneself and one's world (Panzarella et al. 2006), which can contribute to cognitive components of resilience, including maintaining optimism and positive self-regard. A supportive social network can also aid in encouraging active, adaptive coping behavior. People may be more inclined to minimize the appraisal of threat and to act in their own best interests if they perceive a safety net in their social networks. Social support networks can include family, friends, coworkers, mentors and role models, spiritual or religious leaders, and others. Cultivating and nurturing these relationships to form a strong and enduring social support network can be an invaluable means of promoting resilience in the face of trauma. Clinicians should talk with patients about the people in their lives and around them and help them identify opportunities to reach out to establish connections. Patients should be encouraged to reach out to those people who might be most willing to receive them or be able to offer help. Online forums such as Meetup and other interest-based groups can be resources for opportunities to meet like-minded others. Support groups or other resources may also exist, and the clinician should direct patients to these resources and encourage that they follow through.

Face Fears Instead of Avoiding Them

Often, a person's first response to a situation that induces fear or anxiety is to try as hard as possible to avoid the situation and to minimize the experience of fear. Fear is an adaptive human experience meant to inform people about potential danger in the environment. Although it is important to listen to this emotion to identify truly dangerous situations, it is also important to acknowledge that avoidance should not be an automatic reaction. Indeed, some psychiatric disorders are conceptualized, in part, in terms of nonacceptance of the experience of fear and maladaptive efforts to avoid fear, anxiety, or uncertainty (e.g., Hayes et al. 1996). Accepting the experience of fear and anxiety and pushing oneself to face fears can help promote resilience when one experiences subsequent traumatic experiences.

Stress inoculation, involving prior exposure to manageable stressors, has been shown to reduce the behavioral and physiological responses to subsequent stressors (Meichenbaum 1996). By increasing one's sense of control and mastery of stressful situations and by reducing the amount of anxiety experienced when confronted with a stressful or traumatic situation, one can learn to respond more adaptively. Practice with facing fears provides opportunities for stress inoculation, learning to cope with fear actively and adaptively, and possibly increasing one's self-esteem. In light of this, the clinician would do well to investigate previous experiences the patient has had with successfully confronting fears and can help enhance this factor by identifying with the patient new opportunities to face his or her fears. The clinician should be careful to recommend exposure only to feared situations that the patient is likely to be able to tolerate and to work with the patient beforehand to instill skills, such as relaxation and mindfulness, to increase the likelihood of successfully tolerating the distress during exposure. After a few successful experiences of tolerating distress associated with feared situations, the patient might begin to consider the possibility that he or she can successfully tolerate the distress associated with his or her trauma as well.

Attend to Physical Well-Being

Establishing a regimen of physical exercise and/or activity can have a number of beneficial effects for a patient. Physical exercise contributes to physical hardiness and the practical ability to physically endure or survive certain situations. Physical activity has been shown to contribute to improved mood and self-esteem, and an emerging body of multidisciplinary literature has documented the beneficial influence of physical activity on aspects of cognition and brain function (Hillman et al. 2008). A growing number of studies support the idea that physical exercise is a lifestyle factor that might lead to increased physical and mental health throughout life. With regard to resilience, physical activity prior to trauma exposure can provide increased self-esteem and optimism about the chances for survival. During and after trauma exposure, physical activity can improve mood and cognitive capacities for emotion regulation and cognitive flexibility. Clinicians should inquire about patients' physical exercise regimens and encourage them to get enough exercise, at a level befitting their physical capabilities. For example, a regimen of walking 30 minutes three times per week is a good minimum regimen for someone who cannot tolerate more rigorous exercise.

Identify, Utilize, and Foster Character Strengths

Each person has relative strengths and weaknesses. One can attempt to identify one's particular character strengths that might contribute to the components of resilience described in the section "What to Look For." These can include character strengths such as extroversion and interpersonal savoir faire, stress (or fear) tolerance, openness to new experiences, sense of humor, trait optimism, and capacities for emotion regulation. These character strengths can be capitalized on in an effort to cultivate the psychosocial factors that will promote resilience to trauma. For example, extroversion is helpful in establishing and nurturing a supportive social network. Openness to new experiences and tolerance of stress or fear can be capitalized on for stress inoculation and facing one's fears. In addition, one can learn to recognize one's character strengths and engage them when confronting and responding to stressful or traumatic situations. Last, identifying one's particular character strengths can help identify areas of relative weaknesses, which one can then attempt to further develop and strengthen. The clinician can discuss with patients what they perceive to be their character strengths—what has gotten them through difficult times before, what others have commended them for or admired about them in the past—and use his or her own interactions with and observations of patients to help identify strengths they are unable (or perhaps unwilling) to acknowledge.

Changing a characteristic or strengthening a specific area takes time and typically involves regular and rigorous training. Change requires systematic and disciplined activity. A clinician can help a patient by collaboratively generating a training plan and checking in with the patient to encourage adherence. Each patient should be encouraged to concentrate on training in multiple areas: emotional intelligence, moral integrity, facing fears, physical endurance, and so forth.

IMPLICATIONS FOR PSYCHOSOCIAL INTERVENTIONS TO PROMOTE RESILIENCE AFTER TRAUMA

Psychosocial interventions to aid people who have experienced trauma can be tailored to promote resilience by targeting the factors described earlier (see section "What to Look For"). Several interventions comprising elements of cognitive-behavioral psychotherapies have already been developed and investigated for patients in whom psychiatric symptoms or disorders emerge after trauma exposure (e.g., PTSD, major depression, substance-related disorders). The two interventions that have received the most empirical support for treating PTSD and associated symptoms are prolonged exposure (PE) and cognitive processing therapy (CPT).

PE (Williams et al. 2010) is a therapy designed to help posttraumatic patients process traumatic events and reduce psychological disturbances. PTSD is characterized by reexperiencing of the traumatic event through intrusive and upsetting memories, nightmares, and flashbacks and by emotional and physiological reactions to reminders of the trauma, and PTSD patients often try to ward off these intrusive symptoms and avoid any potential trauma reminders, which exacerbates their impairment. PE attempts to address these issues by including two core components: imaginal exposure and in vivo exposure. In imaginal exposure, the traumatic memories are revisited and narrated aloud by the patient, enabling him or her to process the revisiting experience. After the patient has had repeated experiences with imaginal exposure, in vivo exposure is introduced. This component involves repeated confrontation with situations and objects that cause distress. Overall, the goal of PE is to promote processing of the trauma memory and thereby reduce the distress experienced and the avoidance behaviors. In this regard, PE maps onto two components of resilience: facing one's fears and minimizing the continued appraisal of threat.

CPT (Resick and Schnicke 1993) conceptualizes PTSD as a disorder of "nonrecovery" fueled by erroneous beliefs about the causes and consequences of the traumatic event. These beliefs result in strong negative emotions and subsequent avoidance of the trauma memory and of situations that trigger reminders. Combined, these prevent adaptive processing of the trauma memory and the emotions emanating from the event. CPT incorporates cognitive techniques to help patients more accurately appraise these "stuck points" and progress toward recovery, with a primary focus on helping patients to confront, gain an understanding of, and modify the meaning attributed to the traumatic events. In the early stage of CPT, patients learn to identify automatic thoughts and maladaptive beliefs about themselves and the trauma and to increase awareness of the relationship between their thoughts and feelings. The next stage of CPT includes formal processing of the trauma, either in writing or in verbal communication with the therapist, to break the pattern of avoidance. In the final stage, patients learn cognitive skills to evaluate and modify their beliefs about themselves and the traumatic events they have experienced and to challenge and reframe their maladaptive conclusions about their traumatic experiences (e.g., that "this means that no one can ever be trusted").

PE and CPT represent the most empirically supported, state-of-the-art cognitive-behavioral therapies for recovering from trauma. Although each technique includes components that map onto some important factors for promoting resilience, the therapist needs to tailor each approach to account for all factors and enhance the patient's ability to engender resilience. Table 9–2 includes examples of cognitive and behavioral psychotherapeutic techniques that can be used to foster the associated psychosocial resilience factors.

PE provides opportunities to engage and practice active coping skills: minimizing the continued appraisal of threat and facing one's fears. CPT provides opportunities to engage these active coping skills, develop cognitive flexibility (reappraising, reframing, and assimilating traumatic experiences; accepting trauma), and embrace a personal moral compass (maintaining adaptive core beliefs, finding meaning in trauma). To enhance these interventions' ability to promote resilience even further, the clinician should address the remaining psychosocial factors. In particular, efforts to cultivate interpersonal relationships and form a supportive social network are absent in PE and CPT. Some intervention strategies, including brief eclectic psychotherapy for PTSD (Gersons et al. 2000), Skills Training in Affective and Interpersonal Regulation (STAIR) Narrative Story Telling (NST; Cloitre et al. 2010), and dialectical behavior therapy (Bohus et al. 2013), explicitly address enhancing interpersonal effectiveness

TABLE 9–2.   **Techniques to facilitate the psychosocial factors underlying resilience**

Factor	Cognitive approaches	Behavioral approaches
Optimism	Normalize experience; modification of core beliefs and expectancies for the future	
Cognitive flexibility	Practice reappraising, reframing, and assimilating life experiences (traumatic and nontraumatic) Cultivate acceptance for distress, difficulties, and so on Develop mindfulness for thoughts and feelings	
Active coping skills	Monitor automatic thoughts Minimize continued appraisal of threat Maintain positive self-regard in the face of adversity	Practice asking for and seeking help and resources Expose to/inoculate against unwanted/aversive thoughts and feelings Practice facing one's fears
Physical health		Engage in behavioral activation: physical activity and exercise
Social support network		Establish and maintain interpersonal relationships Connect with a resilient role model
Personal moral compass	Maintain adaptive, positive core beliefs	Engage in altruistic behavior Engage with faith/spiritual leaders, role models, and so on Engage in activities and goals that yield purpose and meaning for life

and/or cultivating a supportive social network in the treatment and have begun to receive empirical support for the treatment of PTSD. Another approach to addressing this factor could be to pair trauma survivors with mentors or role models who have successfully navigated their own traumatic experiences. Including a behavioral activation component (Jacobson et al. 2001)—which has been shown to be effective in the treatment of depressive disorders (Spates et al. 2006), which often co-occur with PTSD—could also be effective in promoting resilience. Developing behaviors related to physical activity and altruistic or other prosocial behaviors might be particularly effective because they correspond to important psychosocial factors of resilience. Last, encouraging spiritual or religious coping as a means of enhancing faith and optimism for the future as well as purpose in life could be included as components of these expanded interventions. Taken together, these psychotherapeutic approaches to treating trauma survivors have been shown to be effective in reducing PTSD symptoms, and there may be opportunities to expand these interventions to include other psychosocial factors to promote resilience even more.

Resilience-focused training programs are being developed that specifically target the psychosocial factors described in previous sections. These programs aim to develop resilience by training mindfulness and attention so that one becomes more aware of the present moment as opposed to ruminating on the past and the difficult emotions that it engenders. In this way, mindfulness is trained as a means of enhancing emotion regulation. Using purposeful, trained attention, one may decrease the frequency, intensity, and duration of negative thoughts and associated feelings and bring greater focus on the present moment. In addition, these training programs aim to foster acceptance for the stressful or traumatic event, find meaning in life, develop gratitude, and even address spirituality.

Case Vignette

Mr. B is an African American male in his 50s who is employed driving subway trains in a city. Mr. B arrived at the psychiatric emergency room after witnessing a man commit suicide by jumping in front of the subway train he was driving. Mr. B was experiencing acute anxiety and emotional lability after witnessing the death from very close range and reported reexperiencing the painful images he saw and sounds he heard. The clinician probed for Mr. B's thoughts about the event and his plans for returning to work. Mr. B reported that he did not wish to encounter any reminders of what happened and was considering quitting his job so that he could avoid the situation altogether. He also reported a belief that he "should not discuss this with others because it could traumatize them as well."

The clinician identified the following factors as opportunities for Mr. B to cope with the traumatic event and foster resilience: facing his fears instead of avoiding them and relying on a social support network. The clinician also normalized Mr. B's experience of the trauma and the subsequent symptoms he experienced. Mr. B was encouraged not to quit his job but to request a temporary reassignment because he would be unable to drive the subway train again until he felt more at ease. The clinician offered to and ultimately did contact the supervisor to help Mr. B make this request, which was granted. Mr. B was also encouraged to identify others who have experienced traumatic events, to ask them how they coped, and to share his experience with them. Mr. B was hesitant to discuss this situation with his family for fear of traumatizing them, but he did identify a friend and a coworker who had overcome other traumatic situations with whom he was willing to talk. The clinician role-played with Mr. B how he might approach these people to begin this dialogue. Mr. B was ultimately able to connect with them, and they formed a supportive social network outside of his family on which Mr. B relied for several months as he came to terms with what he had experienced. The clinician regularly checked in with Mr. B over the phone to gauge his success reaching out to his friend and coworker and later to encourage him to continue the dialogue when he appeared to distance himself from them. The clinician was also helpful in preparing Mr. B to return to his original job driving the subway train when the time came, by again normalizing the fear and anxiety he experienced and conveying the belief that Mr. B was capable of tolerating the distress while still moving forward with his life.

Case Vignette

Ms. Z is a 28-year-old white woman who was employed in the financial industry prior to the 2008 financial meltdown, in which Ms. Z lost her job. Ms. Z had worked with the same company since graduating from college and had a relatively successful career that she had assumed was secure. When she lost her job, Ms. Z's view of herself and her career changed dramatically. She developed much self-doubt and pessimism about returning to a career she valued. She also developed significant symptoms of anxiety and depression. She withdrew from friends and family, began drinking alcohol excessively, and stopped doing things that she enjoyed.

Ms. Z entered psychotherapy to address these symptoms, and the clinician focused on several psychosocial facets of resilience to enhance. Cognitive-behavioral strategies such as challenging and reframing negative cognitions about herself and the future were used, and she eventually internalized the belief that this experience was not "just me" and began to acknowledge that many others had suffered the same fate. Accordingly, she began to believe that "things can turn around eventually." This fostered optimism instead of pessimism. She was also encouraged to find a resilient role model. She began meeting weekly with a mentor from her industry who had overcome similar career difficulties and was able to share her own coping strategies, validate Ms. Z's distress, and offer hope. This relationship also served to behaviorally activate her and provide a social support. Ms. Z was also encouraged to focus more on her physical activity; she had been an athlete in college but had not been especially active in recent years. She began training for a triathlon with her newfound time, and this provided some meaning and value for her life, in addition to physical exercise. Over time her anxiety and depression lessened and Ms. Z reengaged with family and friends and began to return to her life. She eventually was able to find a new job.

Key Points

- People's reactions to stress and trauma can range from resilience on the one hand to severe psychopathology, including posttraumatic stress disorder, on the other.

- A constellation of factors have been identified that contribute to resilience in response to stress or trauma. These factors include optimism, cognitive flexibility, active coping skills, maintaining a supportive social network, attending to one's physical well-being, and embracing a personal moral compass.

- These factors can be cultivated even before exposure to traumatic events, or they can be targeted in interventions for patients recovering from trauma exposure.

- Currently available interventions that have been developed for patients who have experienced trauma could be expanded to further address these psychosocial factors in an effort to promote resilience.

- Enhancing resilient outcomes requires that clinicians be active and engaged with patients.

SUGGESTED READINGS

Iacoviello BM, Charney DS: Psychosocial facets of resilience: implications for preventing posttrauma psychopathology, treating trauma survivors, and enhancing community resilience. Eur J Psychotraumatol 5:23970, 2014
Southwick SM, Charney DS: Resilience: The Science of Mastering Life's Greatest Challenges. New York, Cambridge University Press, 2012

REFERENCES

Alim TN, Feder A, Graves RE, et al; DS: Trauma, resilience, and recovery in a high-risk African-American population. Am J Psychiatry 165(12):1566–1575, 2008 19015233
Alloy LB, Just N, Panzarella C: Attributional style, daily life events, and hopelessness depression: subtype validation by prospective variability and specificity of symptoms. Cognit Ther Res 21:321–344, 1997
Bohus M, Dyer AS, Priebe K, et al: Dialectical behaviour therapy for post-traumatic stress disorder after childhood sexual abuse in patients with and without borderline personality disorder: a randomised controlled trial. Psychother Psychosom 82(4):221–233, 2013 23712109
Breslau N, Kessler RC, Chilcoat HD, et al: Trauma and posttraumatic stress disorder in the community: the 1996 Detroit Area Survey of Trauma. Arch Gen Psychiatry 55(7):626–632, 1998 9672053
Burns DD: The Feeling Good Handbook: Using the New Mood Therapy in Everyday Life. New York, William Morrow, 1989
Carver CS, Scheier MF, Segerstrom SC: Optimism. Clin Psychol Rev 30(7):879–889, 2010 20170998

Cloitre M, Stovall-McClough KC, Nooner K, et al: Treatment for PTSD related to childhood abuse: a randomized controlled trial. Am J Psychiatry 167(8):915–924, 2010 20595411

Collins J (producer): The Stockdale Paradox: The Brutal Facts. Audio podcast, 2014. Available at: http://www.jimcollins.com/media_topics/brutal-facts.html. Accessed June 19, 2015.

Connor KM, Davidson JRT: Development of a new resilience scale: the Connor-Davidson Resilience Scale (CD-RISC). Depress Anxiety 18(2):76–82, 2003 12964174

Feder A, Nestler EJ, Charney DS: Psychobiology and molecular genetics of resilience. Nat Rev Neurosci 10(6):446–457, 2009 19455174

Gersons BPR, Carlier IVE, Lamberts RD, et al: Randomized clinical trial of brief eclectic psychotherapy for police officers with posttraumatic stress disorder. J Trauma Stress 13(2):333–347, 2000 10838679

Hayes SC, Wilson KG, Gifford EV, et al: Experimental avoidance and behavioral disorders: a functional dimensional approach to diagnosis and treatment. J Consult Clin Psychol 64(6):1152–1168, 1996 8991302

Hillman CH, Erickson KI, Kramer AF: Be smart, exercise your heart: exercise effects on brain and cognition. Nat Rev Neurosci 9(1):58–65, 2008 18094706

Jacobson NS, Martell CR, Dimidjian S: Behavioral activation for depression: returning to contextual roots. Clin Psychol Sci Pract 8:255–270, 2001

Leontopoulou S: An exploratory study of altruism in Greek children: relations with empathy, resilience and classroom climate. Psychology 1:377–385, 2010

Meichenbaum D: Stress inoculation training for coping with stressors. Clin Psychol 49:4–7, 1996

Panzarella C, Alloy L, Whitehouse W: Expanded hopelessness theory of depression: on the mechanisms by which social support protects against depression. Cognit Ther Res 30:307–333, 2006

Pargament KI, Koenig HG, Tarakeshwar N, et al: Religious coping methods as predictors of psychological, physical and spiritual outcomes among medically ill elderly patients: a two-year longitudinal study. J Health Psychol 9(6):713–730, 2004 15367751

Resick PA, Schnicke MK: Cognitive Processing Therapy for Rape Victims: A Treatment Manual. Newbury Park, CA, Sage, 1993

Scully D, Kremer J, Meade MM, et al: Physical exercise and psychological well being: a critical review. Br J Sports Med 32(2):111–120, 1998 9631216

Smith BW, Pargament KI, Brant C, et al: Noah revisited: religious coping and the impact of a flood. J Community Psychol 28:169–186, 2000

Southwick SM, Vythilingam M, Charney DS: The psychobiology of depression and resilience to stress: implications for prevention and treatment. Annu Rev Clin Psychol 1:255–291, 2005 17716089

Spates C, Pagoto S, Kalata A: A qualitative and quantitative review of behavioral activation treatment of major depressive disorder. Behav Analyst Today 7(4):508–518, 2006

Tsai J, Harpaz-Rotem I, Pietrzak RH, et al: The role of coping, resilience, and social support in mediating the relation between PTSD and social functioning in veterans returning from Iraq and Afghanistan. Psychiatry 75(2):135–149, 2012 22642433

Williams M, Cahill S, Foa E: Psychotherapy for posttraumatic stress disorder, in Textbook of Anxiety Disorders, 2nd Edition. Edited by Stein DJ, Hollander E, Rothbaum BO. Washington, DC, American Psychiatric Publishing, 2010, pp 603–627

CHAPTER 10

Medical-Legal Aspects of Trauma- and Stressor- Related Disorders

JAMES J. STRAIN, M.D.
PATRICIA R. CASEY, M.D., F.R.C.PSYCH.
PHILLIP J. RESNICK, M.D.
HENRY C. WEINSTEIN, M.D.

PSYCHIATRISTS WORKING with trauma- and stressor-related disorders frequently encounter clinical situations that have legal implications. This group of disorders is a touchstone for many of the broader challenges that arise in psychiatry, and in this chapter we discuss the common legal issues faced by psychiatrists in this context. These include capacity evaluations, informed consent, confidentiality, dual loyalty, malingering, the use of questionnaires, and the role of the psychiatrist as a witness in court proceedings.

The American Academy of Psychiatry and the Law (2005) defines *forensic psychiatry* as "a subspecialty of psychiatry in which scientific and clinical expertise is applied in legal contexts involving civil, criminal, correctional, regulatory or legislative matters, and in specialized clinical consultations in areas such as risk assessment or employment." To begin, legal matters are broadly separated into civil matters and criminal matters. The rules that apply and the roles of the parties are quite different in these two contexts. Civil matters, such as torts, generally involve only money, whereas criminal matters may threaten a person's liberty and result in incarceration in a correctional facility.

COMPETENCE AND CONSENT

The most common legal question in psychiatry is the question of *competence* (also referred to as *capacity*). This is defined as the degree of mental soundness necessary to make decisions (about a specific issue). It is important to note that clinicians can determine capacity, but only a court or judge can determine competency.

Competence is an issue that impinges on every psychiatrist, and all adults are assumed to have competence unless adjudged otherwise. Competence assessments may arise in the context of making wills and in making major decisions such as getting married or selling a house. In clinical practice competence is most frequently relevant in relation to consent to treatment.

The concept of informed consent is anchored in the principle articulated by Justice Benjamin Cardozo: "Every human being of adult years and sound mind has a right to determine what shall be done with his own body" (*Schloendorff v. Society of New York Hospital* 1914). Physicians tend to question a patient's capacity to consent if the patient makes what is viewed by the physicians as the "wrong" decision. The test of competence, in principle, is independent of the choice made; however, in practice, the test of competence is often linked to the risk-benefit analysis of the decision. For example, if the risk-benefit ratio of treatment is favorable, a low test of competence is employed if the patient consents and a high standard of competence if the patient refuses. If the risk-benefit ratio of treatment is unfavorable, a high test of competence is employed if the patient consents and a lower test if the patient refuses. For example, if a person with severe posttraumatic stress disorder (PTSD) refuses eye movement desensitization and reprocessing treatment, for which a risk-benefit ratio of treatment is favorable, a high test of competence is employed; if the patient agrees, then a lower standard of competence is used.

Competence assessments are carried out routinely when patients refuse treatment or when they seek to discharge themselves from the hospital against medical advice. Although any licensed physician may make a determination of capacity, a physician frequently calls a psychiatrist for the evaluation if there is uncertainty about the person's ability to consent to a medically indicated treatment.

In the context of trauma- and stressor-related disorders, questions of competence may arise in a variety of cases. For example, an evaluation may be requested when a patient with cancer, diagnosed with an adjustment disorder because of extreme distress at the diagnosis, is refusing chemotherapy. Likewise, a person with PTSD who refuses to engage with treatment because of concerns about reexperiencing the trauma during sessions may be subject to a competence evaluation. Frequently, a patient's refusal to accept medical treatment stems from poor understanding of the proposed treatment; therefore, a careful explanation must be a prerequisite to any such assessment.

Competence assessments are narrowly focused and refer only to the issue at hand. The fact that a person lacks capacity in one area does not imply a lack in others. For instance, a person who lacks capacity to make a treatment decision may have the capacity to make a will. With regard to the treatment decision, it is necessary that the patient fully understand what is being said to him or her and that he or she can retain the information. Capacity can fluctuate with the state of the patient (e.g., during an acute confusional state, capacity will be impaired but will likely improve once the condition has resolved unless there is an underlying dementia).

Voluntariness

Consent to treatment (or to any other aspect of life, such as marriage) must be voluntary; that is, a patient's decision should be made according to his or her own free will, without constraint or expectation of reward. Attention should be paid to the relationship between an individual's decision and the influence of loved ones. Consent is not voluntary when a loved one, such as a spouse or parent, is excessively influencing the patient. An exception to this rule is minors, who depend on adult decision makers. Decisions made under duress or as a result of unrealistic fears are not truly voluntary. When a patient cannot choose among alternatives because of his or her irrational fears, free choice is impaired. Some fear might be within normal range and dissipate once an explanation is offered. At other times the fear may be appropriate to the situation, but if a patient is influenced or impaired by paranoia or other psychotic thinking or by major depression (i.e., feeling that he or she is worthless), then free choice would be considered to be impaired.

Information

Informed consent requires an understanding of the following: 1) the medical-psychiatric condition, 2) the nature and effect of the proposed treatment, 3) the risks and benefits of the treatment, 4) the likely result of refusal, and 5) alternative treatments. It is important to ensure that the patient demonstrates an understanding of his or her condition. What appears to be a lack of decision-making capacity may in fact be the result of a communication barrier, and this possibility must be carefully evaluated in those who do not speak the language sufficiently well to understand the information given. Patients with a learning disorder may also have impaired understanding.

Exceptions to Informed Consent

Courts recognize the following four exceptions to informed consent:

1. *Emergency:* Treatment may be delivered without consent to a patient who is unconscious or in imminent danger of serious harm. Most physicians are aware of this exception and are comfortable proceeding with treatment in the absence of a psychiatric consultation. There may be times when a psychiatrist will need to inform the medical team that they can proceed in an emergency.
2. *Incompetence:* Incompetent patients, by definition, cannot give informed consent. In such a case, consent should be obtained from a guardian or substitute decision maker. Typically, it is the consultant's opinion regarding the patient's inability to make medical decisions that results in a determination of incompetence (lack of capacity).
3. *Waiver:* A patient may waive his or her right to receive information. For example, a patient may tell the doctor, "Don't tell me what's happening; just do what you think is best." Thus, the patient is accepting the doctor's decision to make unilateral medical decisions. A waiver is valid if the patient is competent (or has capacity) to waive disclosure and the decision is documented in the medical record. As part of the assessment of competence in these circumstances, the doctor should list the reasons for the waiver.
4. *Therapeutic privilege:* A doctor may decide to withhold information from a patient because telling that information would cause psychological damage or render the patient ineffective in decision making. Therapeutic privilege is a narrowly defined exception to informed consent. If a clinical situation warrants therapeutic privilege, the doctor must make disclosure to a relative as an alternative to secure consent and document the reason for this clinical decision. This situation is unlikely to arise in relation to trauma- and stressor-related disorders but is included here for completeness.

Tests and Questionnaires to Assist in Competence Assessments

MacArthur Competence Assessment Tool-Treatment

The MacArthur Competence Assessment Tool-Treatment (MacCAT-T; Grisso and Appelbaum 1998) is an interviewing tool used to evaluate a patient's decision-making abilities. The MacCAT-T's design was modeled on the data collected in the MacArthur Treatment Competence Study (Appelbaum and Grisso

1995). The MacCAT-T is the most frequently used screening tool to evaluate patients' decision-making capacities.

The MacArthur Treatment Competence Study was designed to provide information to policy makers and clinicians to help them address questions about the decision-making capacities of people who are hospitalized with mental illness. The four legally relevant abilities addressed were (Appelbaum and Grisso 1995)

1. the ability to state a choice
2. the ability to understand relevant information
3. the ability to appreciate the nature of one's own situation
4. the ability to reason about the potential risks and benefits

Mini-Mental Status Examination

The Mini-Mental State Examination (MMSE; Folstein et al. 1975) is a routine examination conducted for the purpose of cognitive screening. Kim and Caine (2002) examined the utility and the limits of the MMSE in capacity evaluations and concluded that the MMSE was limited in its ability to measure decisional capacity. An MMSE score of 26 or less has a sensitivity of 91%–99% in identifying persons who are incapable of providing consent, and an MMSE score of 19 or less has a specificity range of 85%–94% for identifying individuals likely to be deemed incapable of providing consent (Kim et al. 2002).

LITIGATION

Witness of Fact and Expert Witness

In the context of litigation involving the trauma- and stressor-related disorders, the psychiatrist may be called to give evidence. The two circumstances in which this occurs are when the psychiatrist is treating the patient and when a psychiatrist is retained by an attorney as an independent expert.

A psychiatrist is a *witness of fact* when he or she has factual knowledge of the patient from work as the person's treating doctor. The evidence must be confined to the facts of the case that are known.

An *expert witness* is a person who by virtue of his or her knowledge and expertise is in a position to assist the judge (and jury if there is one) in understanding the technical or scientific issues at hand. This role is much broader than that of the witness of fact. The role of the expert is governed by the Federal Rules of Evidence in the majority of U.S. states. These rules do not formally define the duties of an expert witness or contain any specific written obligation for the expert to be independent. In this regard they differ from practice in the United Kingdom, where there is a requirement to include a declaration in the report that the opinion is independent and is not determined by who is instructing the expert. In Ireland there is no such requirement, but it is now becoming customary to include such a declaration also. According to the American Academy of Psychiatry and the Law (2005), "Psychiatrists should not distort their opinion in the service of the retaining party."

The expert will usually be expected to interview the litigant as part of the assessment, but in some types of cases (e.g., malpractice or negligence cases in which suicide has occurred), a personal examination is not feasible or required. In other forensic evaluations, if, after appropriate effort, it is not possible to conduct a personal examination, an opinion may nonetheless be rendered on the basis of other information; however, the absence of a personal examination must be clearly indicated in the report.

Rule 29 of the U.S. Federal Rules of Civil Procedure allows for the pretrial taking of evidence in the form of an oral (Rule 30) or written (Rule 31) deposition. The use of a deposition is an important component of *discovery* (the right to compel an opposing party to disclose facts and documents supporting its position) in the U.S. legal system because it enables lawyers to determine the strength of the other side's evidence and therefore may facilitate an early settlement or guide trial tactics. In the United Kingdom and Ireland, reports are exchanged between sides, but oral depositions are not part of the legal process. However, in the United Kingdom expert witnesses meet in advance of the trial to decide on areas of difference and agreement. The trial will hear those elements for which there are unresolvable disagreements.

A commonly asked question is how medical experts can disagree if they are basing their opinion on science. Is it possible that one expert is a "hired gun?" This is a consideration, but such a situation will usually become obvious during cross-examination if the evaluation has been distorted or deliberately skewed. Provided that both experts form their opinion in good faith, this will not be an issue. Even in day-to-day clinical practice, doctors disagree about the best way to manage individual patients.

Confidentiality and Dual Loyalty

Confidentiality is the cornerstone of the doctor-patient relationship, and the exceptions to it are discussed in the next subsection, "Confidentiality and the Legal Process". An important consideration is what constitutes best practice when situations of dual loyalty arise. An example of such a situation is when a hospital manager requests that one of the staff psychiatrists evaluate a staff member who has an unacceptable level of absenteeism to find out whether the person has a psychiatric illness that requires treatment. At the outset the psychiatrist should clarify to the evaluee for whom the psychiatrist is conducting the examination and what will be done with the information obtained. At the beginning of a forensic evaluation, care should be taken to explicitly inform the evaluee that the psychiatrist is not the evaluee's "doctor." Psychiatrists have a continuing obligation to be sensitive to the fact that although a warning has been given, the evaluee may develop the belief that there is a treatment relationship. If the patient requires treatment, he or she should be referred to another psychiatrist, but if this is not possible, the evaluee should be advised that the employer may request progress reports. Psychiatrists should take precautions to ensure that only necessary information is released and that they do not release confidential information to unauthorized persons. Medical information should be released to other medical professionals only if legally mandated.

Confidentiality and the Legal Process

Important questions often present in relation to confidentiality and the legal process: How does the principle of confidentiality comport with the necessity to prepare patient reports that will be disseminated to nonmedical professionals and become public when introduced in court? What are doctors' duties and responsibilities when asked to provide such information? Can a doctor refuse?

Both the American Medical Association and the American Psychiatric Association (APA) have adopted codes of ethics that specify practitioners' ethical responsibility to maintain confidentiality. The federal Health Insurance Portability and Accountability Act of 1996 (HIPAA) also includes a confidentiality provision. The concept of confidentiality can be traced back to the Hippocratic Oath. The concept of doctor-patient privilege refers to the patient's right to prevent a physician from releasing personal medical information to third parties. Information gained in confidence about a patient may not be released without the authorization of the patient. However, there are exceptions that arise both clinically and legally, particularly in relation to patients with diagnoses in the trauma- and stressor-related group of disorders. Patients need to be aware of the limits of confidentiality. When a clinician is breaching confidentiality ethically, only information that is relevant to a given situation or question should be disclosed.

Clinical Exceptions to Confidentiality

Information about a patient may be released without the individual's consent when it is necessary to protect that person in an emergency, as in this example: A patient presents to the emergency room with a complaint of depression and feeling hopeless following a recent bereavement. The patient denies feeling suicidal; however, the patient's history is significant for two previous suicide attempts. The patient insists on being discharged to go home. The patient cannot forbid the physician from contacting relatives to ascertain information necessary to assess the suicide risk.

The consultant may also breach confidentiality if another person is in danger. For example, an adult with complex PTSD who reports having been sexually abused as a child should be advised of the requirement to report the perpetrator if that person is still alive. Elder abuse and infectious diseases must also be reported to the relevant authorities. According to the APA position statement, reporting of HIV to a third party who is not at ongoing risk may still be beneficial because doing so may allow for the identification of infection before the onset of clinical symptoms. However, states' regulations regarding the physician's duty to report HIV infection to a third party vary and may differ from positions taken by national organizations. Therefore, it is important for psychiatric consultants to review the regulations in the state in which they practice and to seek consultation with the hospital attorney as necessary.

The following case is an example of this exception to patient confidentiality.

Case Vignette

Mr. M, a 35-year-old single bus driver, was admitted to a psychiatric unit following a serious overdose after the death of his mother 3 weeks earlier. He was diagnosed with an adjustment disorder. He was tearful and irritable throughout the admission and asked to leave the hospital "as soon as possible.... I have to be back at work." In the course of the psychiatric evaluation, Mr. M admitted to binge drinking, although he had previously denied substance use. He confided, "I haven't been up front with everyone about my drinking. I don't want to lose my job.... It's the only income I've got." When questioned about drinking on the job, he denied using alcohol during the week (he works on weekdays). The psychiatric consultant provided a referral for substance abuse counseling. Mr. M agreed to substance abuse counseling, emphatically denied that he would drink again, and demanded that the psychiatric consultant "keep this confidential."

Discussion: As a school bus driver using alcohol excessively, Mr. M puts children at risk by virtue of his excessive alcohol use. Despite Mr. M's denial of using alcohol on the job and agreement to pursue substance abuse treatment, the psychiatric consultant has a duty to disclose this to his employer. This duty is mandated by the code of ethics outlined by the APA. The employer may then mandate ongoing substance abuse treatment and monitoring as a condition of employment. The psychiatric consultant may be subject to disciplinary action if the impaired employee is not reported to the employer.

If a patient poses a threat to the life of another, the person under threat and/ or the police should be notified. This is known as a *Tarasoff* warning after a case against the University of California in 1974 in which a therapist at the university failed to warn Tatiana Tarasoff that her former boyfriend, a patient of the therapist's, was threatening to kill her. When he did kill her, Ms. Tarasoff's parents successfully sued the university (*Tarasoff v. Regents of the University of California*). Some jurisdictions now require not only that the victim should be warned but also that the doctor has a general duty to protect the intended victim. Advice on how to issue such a warning should be sought from the hospital lawyer.

Exceptions to Confidentiality Governed by Law or the Courts

The forensic consideration arises when psychiatrists are asked to provide reports to the court regarding patients with trauma- or stressor-related disorders who decide to sue those they believe to have been responsible for the triggering events. Compensation may be sought from an agency such as the army when, for example, individuals are injured in the course of service abroad. No organization or individual is exempt from litigation for being negligent with respect to employees. It might be an insurance company that provides coverage to the owner of a vehicle involved in a traffic accident or an individual who has bullied another.

There are five exceptions to the rule of confidentiality in these circumstances. Reports to the court, prepared by a psychiatrist serving as a witness of fact (i.e., the treating psychiatrist) or an expert witness (i.e., an independent expert employed by either the plaintiff or the defense), represent the first two exceptions to the confidentiality rule. This is because all relevant material disclosed by the patient must be included in the report and may be revealed in a public court.

The third exception is when a judge orders the patient's medical records to be provided to the defendants. This release is often done by voluntary agreement, but discovery may be ordered, also by a judge. When the notes are being released, the names of all persons other than the litigant/plaintiff/defendant should be redacted from the records, as should any information not relevant to the specific issue at hand. For example, in a case involving a claim for PTSD following an accident, information from the patient's spouse that he (the spouse) has been unfaithful would be redacted if it had no bearing on the case. On the other hand, if a woman diagnosed with delusional disorder is suing for misdiagnosis, information disclosed about spousal infidelity by the defendant is germane and should remain.

The fourth exception occurs when the doctor is giving evidence in commitment proceedings and treatment refusal hearings, although in these circumstances the disclosure is to only a few people, who themselves are bound by confidentiality.

The fifth exception applies to individuals on parole, probation, or conditional release or in other custodial or mandatory settings, when failure to adhere to an agreed-on arrangement with the psychiatrist may be reported to legal authorities mandating it.

Levels of Proof

The witness going to court needs to be aware of the level of proof required in a particular case. *Level of proof* is defined as the probability or certainty that the proposition being tested is true (e.g., that the accident caused the disorder claimed or that the person is guilty of the offense with which he is charged). The doctor under cross-examination might therefore be asked probability questions. The following hypothetical case is presented as an example.

Case Vignette

Mr. K experienced an adjustment disorder after his wallet was stolen from his locker at work. He had previously received the same diagnosis when he took an overdose after his marriage broke up. He sued his employer for his mental health problem, claiming that the employer did not take adequate precautions to ensure the safety of the employees.

The doctor giving evidence in this case might be asked, "Given his prior diagnosis, what would the chances be of the plaintiff's having a recurrence of his adjustment disorder if he hadn't been exposed to the stress of his wallet being stolen at work?" Although questions such as this are extremely difficult to answer, the legal teams persist in raising them. A question similar to this is necessary to establish whether the required threshold of proof is reached—for example, 50% or more chance of having a recurrence (see proof level 1 below).

There are three levels of proof:

1. *A preponderance of the evidence,* known also as the *balance of probabilities,* is the standard required in most civil cases (e.g., when a person sues another for damages). It is also the level required in family court determinations solely involving money, such as child support. The standard is met if the proposition is more likely to be true than not true. Effectively, the standard is satisfied if there is a greater than 50% chance that the proposition is true or if it is "more probable than not."
2. *Clear and convincing evidence* requires that the evidence presented by a party during the trial is highly and substantially more probable to be true than not and that the trier of fact has a firm belief or conviction in its factuality. In this standard, a greater degree of believability must be met than the preponderance standard of proof in civil actions. This level of proof is required in cases of civil commitment of patients with mental illness, where an individual's liberty is at stake. An analogous example is a prisoner seeking habeas corpus relief from capital punishment who must prove his factual innocence by clear and convincing evidence. The clear and convincing standard is employed in administrative court determinations, as well as in civil and certain criminal procedures in the United States. This standard is also used in many types of cases, including paternity cases, persons in need of supervision, juvenile delinquency, and child custody; in the probate of wills and living wills; and in petitions to remove a person from life support ("right-to-die" cases). This second level of proof is not used in the United

Kingdom or Ireland, where the balance of probabilities (proof level 1) is applied in all civil cases and the beyond reasonable doubt standard (proof level 3 below) is applied in criminal trials.

3. *Beyond reasonable doubt* is the highest standard used in Anglo-American law and typically applies only in criminal proceedings. It has been described, in negative terms, as a proof having been met if there is no plausible reason to believe otherwise. If there is a real doubt, based on reason and common sense after careful and impartial consideration of all the evidence, or lack of evidence, in a case, then the level of proof has not been met.

It has been said that proof beyond a reasonable doubt is proof of such a convincing character that one would be willing to rely and act on it without hesitation in the most important of one's own affairs. However, it does not mean "with absolute certainty." Judges and justices apply these standards, but physicians testify to a reasonable degree of medical certainty. In most jurisdictions this simply means more likely than not.

MALINGERING

Malingering is more relevant in forensic settings than in day-to-day clinical practice. It should be considered by evaluators involved in the assessment and management of individuals with any of the trauma- and stressor-related disorders. *Malingering* is defined as the conscious fabrication or exaggeration of symptoms or the false imputing of causes that have no relationship to the symptoms for the purposes of external gain. According to a survey of members of the American Board of Clinical Neuropsychology representing 33,531 cases, 29% of personal injury, 30% of disability, 19% of criminal, and 8% of medical cases involved probable malingering and symptom exaggeration (Mittenberg et al. 2002). Malingering has been facilitated by the ease of access to the Internet, where detailed descriptions of symptoms and disorders are widely available. All of the trauma- and stressor-related disorders are potentially open to being malingered because of the subjective nature of the symptoms.

Malingering presents complex problems for an evaluator. A mistaken diagnosis of malingering calls into question the honesty and good name of the person involved and deprives him or her of a just settlement and appropriate treatment. However, failure to identify illness deception leads to unjust financial penalties on the defendant in the case.

In DSM-5 (American Psychiatric Association 2013), malingering receives a V code as a condition that may be a focus of clinical attention. DSM-5 describes malingering as follows:

The essential feature of malingering is the intentional production of false or grossly exaggerated physical or psychological symptoms, motivated by external incentives such as avoiding military duty, avoiding work, obtaining financial compensation, evading criminal prosecution, or obtaining drugs. (p. 726)

One potential barrier to identifying malingering is a doctor's desire to be supportive of the patient. The doctor may simply be reluctant to consider the possibility of malingering because deliberate deception is anathema to the trust that is central to the doctor-patient relationship. This reluctance carries over into the forensic setting, even when doctors are appointed as independent expert witnesses.

Popular misconceptions abound in relation to the detection of lying. For example, paying attention to gaze avoidance, fidgeting, and delay in responding to questions, among other behaviors, is incorrectly believed to assist in the detection of lying. There is no single giveaway clue (like Pinocchio's nose). It is also mistakenly believed that mental health professionals are uniquely capable of detecting when patients are lying. A meta-analysis of 193 studies revealed that psychologists were only marginally better at recognizing lying than student research participants (Aamodt and Custer 2006). Another study (Vrij and Mann 2003) found that there was no evidence that the ability to accurately identify persons who were lying was related to age, sex, or experience. In general, good detectors used different cues for different people rather than adhering to simple rules of thumb. For example, speech cues might be important for detecting lying in some people, whereas body movements or eye movements might be more useful for others.

Many clinicians are unaware of methods that are useful for detecting malingering (conscious fabrication or exaggeration). Some basic approaches are listed in Table 10–1.

Interviewing style is also important (Resnick and Knoll 2005) because there is a danger that the clinician will suggest responses in the phrasing of the prompts or questions. Using open-ended rather than closed questions is the approach least likely to suggest responses. For example, saying "Tell me about your sleep" is preferable to asking "Do you get nightmares?"

A number of questionnaires are used to assist the clinician in the detection of malingering, and a few are summarized here. On the Minnesota Multiphasic Personality Inventory—2 (MMPI-2; Butcher et al. 1989), the F scale identifies symptoms that the public considers to be associated with psychopathology but that are not often found in those with serious psychopathology. The 172-item Structured Interview of Reported Symptoms (SIRS; Rogers et al. 1991) was designed to assess a wide range of psychopathology, particularly psychosis. The SIRS takes about 40 minutes to administer. The Test of Memory Malingering (TOMM; Tombaugh 1997) is a 50-item recognition test for feigned memory,

---

TABLE 10–1.   Diagnosing malingering in clinical practice

1. Consider the possibility of malingering.

2. Check collateral information from independent sources (e.g., family doctor records) to check that the background is presented accurately.

3. Observe the patient when he or she is unaware of being observed, during a period of inpatient assessment if necessary.

4. Obtain video footage if available.

5. Check medication records to confirm claims that medications were prescribed for symptoms related to the incident being considered.

6. Observe whether the patient becomes distressed when speaking about the incident.

7. Observe whether symptoms are consistent during the visit and over time.

8. Assess whether a discrepancy exists between the level of symptoms described and the patient's "functioning."

9. Observe whether the patient becomes defensive in describing past or personal history.

10. Consider whether the patient adheres to treatment and attends appointments.

11. Note whether the patient consents to release of medical records and to the provision of independent collateral information.

12. Ask about improbable symptoms.

13. Use tests and questionnaires as an adjunct, albeit with caution.

---

and the Structured Inventory of Malingered Symptomatology (SIMS) is a 75-item true-or-false screening instrument that assesses both malingered psychopathology and neuropsychological symptoms (Smith and Burger 1997). For a fuller list see Conroy and Kwartner (2006). However, as Drob et al. (2009) point out, these tools do not distinguish between malingering and conditions such as factitious disorder, conversion, or somatoform disorders.

Although malingering is one explanation for unusual symptoms or presentations, there are other explanations that must be borne in mind. If malingering is suspected, there is a possibility that the symptoms are iatrogenic, rather than feigned, due to the reinforcing effects of litigation on symptoms. Alternatively, there may be elements of iatrogenesis due to multiple interviews and frequent testing and conscious symptom exaggeration when there is the possibility of financial reward.

MEMORY IN TRAUMA- AND STRESSOR-RELATED DISORDERS

The diagnosis of trauma- and stressor-related disorders is based on the presence of a stressor that precedes the onset of symptoms. Information on timing is usually dependent on the person's recall of events and on his or her description of symptoms. Although patients may describe particular events, this process can be influenced by several biases. *Recall bias* relates to differences in the ways exposure information is remembered by patients who have experienced an adverse outcome compared with control subjects who have not (Hennekens and Buring 1987). *Attribution bias* is defined as attributing some outcome to a particular event when it may have been caused by another temporally related event (Heider 1958). The current emotional state of the person may also affect recall; if distressed, the person may focus selectively on negative rather than positive experiences, leading to cognitive distortions, also known as negative cognitive bias.

For these reasons, obtaining independent collateral information about events, their timing, and their temporal relationship to symptoms is crucial when a clinician is asked to evaluate causality. Accessing prior medical records and consulting with doctors previously involved in the person's care are critical to making an accurate diagnosis. It is not enough to simply rely on what a patient describes. Normal forgetting, recall bias, and attribution bias can all distort the history.

A study by Southwick et al. (1997) pointed to the unreliability of memory in patients with PTSD. In this study recollections of combat trauma were found to be inconsistent among returned Gulf War veterans, with more memories being recalled at 2-year follow-up than at 1 month after return. Between the two time points, 88% of subjects changed their responses on at least one of the 19 trauma questionnaire items, and 61% changed responses on two or more items. Memory amplification was also associated with greater levels of symptomatology. The authors concluded, "This study raises questions not only about the accuracy of memory for traumatic events, but also about the relationship between traumatic stressors and PTSD" (p. 176). These findings point once again to the problems of memory when assessing issues of causation in this group of disorders.

CAUSATION

Legal causation is an issue for the court to determine, and this will influence the award for injuries sustained. Did the traffic accident in which a woman was involved cause her to develop PTSD symptoms, or was it some other event? What was the role of the sexual abuse she suffered as a child in determining her current symptoms? Does her heavy consumption of alcohol contribute to her symptoms? These are examples of the types of questions that arise in determining the contribution of a specific event to a particular outcome.

Causation is established when the plaintiff proves to the civil standard (a preponderance of the evidence) that the defendant caused or contributed to the injury. The general, but not conclusive, test for causation is the "but for" test, which requires the plaintiff to show that the injury would not have occurred but for the negligence of the defendant. The principle is that the law does not excuse a defendant from liability merely because other causal (background) factors for which he or she is not responsible also helped produce the harm. It is sufficient if the defendant's negligence was a cause of the harm. This is known as the eggshell skull rule. Other less well known rules are the crumbling skull and the old soldier's rules.

The Eggshell Skull or Thin Skull Rule

A very interesting doctrine in the law is known as the eggshell skull rule (or thin skull rule or "take your victim as you find him" rule of the common law). It is a very well established legal doctrine that is used in some tort law systems, and a similar doctrine is applicable to criminal law. This rule holds one liable for all consequences resulting from the negligent actions leading to the injury of another person, even if the victim suffers from a preexisting vulnerability such as a medical condition.

The term implies that if a person had a skull as vulnerable as that of an eggshell and a tortfeasor (wrongdoer) who was unaware of the condition injured that person's head, causing the skull to break unexpectedly, the defendant would be held liable for all damages resulting from the wrongful contact even if he or she did not intend to cause such a severe injury. In other words, but for the tort, the condition of the person would have remained stable.

The same maxim applies in criminal law. There is no requirement of physical contact with the victim. For example, if a trespasser's wrongful presence on the victim's property so terrifies the victim that she has a fatal heart attack, the trespasser will be liable for the damages stemming from his original wrongdoing.

The Crumbling Skull Rule

The eggshell skull rule is not to be confused with the related crumbling skull rule, in which the plaintiff suffers from an aggressive condition (from a prior injury or disease) before the occurrence of the present tort. According to the crumbling skull rule, the prior condition is to be considered only with respect to distinguishing it from any new injury arising from the present tort—as a means of apportioning damages fairly. For example, if a person with continuing PTSD is retraumatized, the tortfeasor has to pay damages only for the additional portion caused by him. On the other hand, if the person had a prior history of PTSD that had become stable and "but for" the litigated accident would have remained so, the eggshell principle would apply and the tortfeasor is fully responsible for the recurrence of symptoms despite the prior vulnerability.

The Old Soldier's Rule

Another principle of tort law, the old soldier's rule, states that a party who harms another will be fully liable for aggravation of a prior injury. For example, if a patient with PTSD has a recurrence following a vehicular accident caused by a drunk driver and then takes his own life and that of his child as a consequence of the accompanying depression, the tortfeasor (the drunk driver) becomes responsible for both deaths.

CONCLUSION

Most psychiatrists will be called on to make decisions that have legal implications, commonly relating to informed consent and capacity. They are also likely to be called as witnesses of fact in the context of their own patients who embark on litigation. Expert witness roles are more specific and apply only to a limited number of clinicians.

Key Points

- A person's competence to make decisions is assumed.

- The psychiatrist must explain dual loyalty to the patient before gathering information.

- Informed consent can be bypassed in certain circumstances.

- Requirements for confidentiality have been codified by the American Psychiatric Association's code of ethics and by the Health Insurance Portability and Accountability Act (HIPAA) in the United States.

- Confidentiality is not absolute, and there are exceptions.

- Psychiatrists may be called as witnesses of fact or as expert witnesses in legal proceedings.

- In the context of litigation, three levels of proof exist: preponderance of evidence, clear and convincing evidence, and beyond reasonable doubt.

- Demonstrating causality between events and outcomes is challenging.

SUGGESTED READINGS

American Academy of Psychiatry and the Law: Ethics Guidelines for the Practice of Forensic Psychiatry. 2005. Available at: www.aapl.org/ethics.htm. Accessed June 20, 2015.

Lowenstein LF: Recent research into dealing with the problem of malingering. Med Leg J 70(Pt 1):38–49, 2002 11915575

REFERENCES

Aamodt MG, Custer H: Who can best catch a liar?—a meta-analysis of individual differences in detecting deception. Forensic Exam 15:6–11, 2006

American Academy of Psychiatry and the Law: Ethics Guidelines for the Practice of Forensic Psychiatry. 2005. Available at: http://www.aapl.org/ethics.htm. Accessed June 20, 2015.

American Psychiatric Association: Diagnostic and Statistical Manual of Mental Disorders, 5th Edition. Arlington, VA, American Psychiatric Association, 2013

Appelbaum PS, Grisso T: The MacArthur Treatment Competence Study, I: mental illness and competence to consent to treatment. Law Hum Behav 19(2):105–126, 1995 11660290

Butcher JN, Williams CL, Graham JR, et al: Minnesota Multiphasic Personality Inventory—2: Manual for Administration and Scoring. Minneapolis, MN, University of Minnesota Press, 1989

Conroy MA, Kwartner PP: Malingering. Applied Psychology in Criminal Justice 2(3):29–51, 2006

Drob SL, Meehan KB, Waxman SE: Clinical and conceptual problems in the attribution of malingering in forensic evaluations. J Am Acad Psychiatry Law 37:98–106, 2009

Folstein MF, Folstein SE, McHugh PR: "Mini-mental state": a practical method for grading the cognitive state of patients for the clinician. J Psychiatr Res 12:189–198, 1975 1202204

Grisso T, Appelbaum PS: MacArthur Competence Assessment Tool for Treatment. Sarasota, FL, Professional Resource Press, 1998

Heider F: The Psychology of Interpersonal Relations. New York, Wiley, 1958

Hennekens CH, Buring JE: Epidemiology in Medicine. Philadelphia, PA, Lippincott Williams & Wilkins, 1987

Kim SY, Caine ED: Utility and limits of the Mini Mental State Examination in evaluating consent capacity in Alzheimer's disease. Psychiatr Serv 53(10):1322–1324, 2002 12364686

Kim SY, Karlawish JH, Caine ED: Current state of research on decision-making competence of cognitively impaired elderly persons. Am J Geriatr Psychiatry 10(2):151–
   165, 2002 11925276
Mittenberg W, Patton C, Canyock EM, et al: Base rates of malingering and symptom ex-
   aggeration. J Clin Exp Neuropsychol 24(8):1094–1102, 2002 12650234
Resnick PJ, Knoll J: Faking it: how to detect malingered psychosis. Current Psychiatry
   4(11):13–25, 2005
Rogers R, Gillis JR, Bagby RM, et al: Detection of malingering on the Structured Interview of Reported Symptoms (SIRS): a study of coached and uncoached simulators.
   Psychol Assess 3(4):673–677, 1991
Schloendorff v Society of New York Hospital, 105 NE 92,93. (1914)
Smith GP, Burger GK: Detection of malingering: validation of the Structured Inventory
   of Malingered Symptomatology (SIMS). Bull Am Acad Psychiatry Law 25:183–189,
   1997 9213290
Southwick SM, Morgan CA 3rd, Nicolaou AL, et al: Consistency of memory for combat-
   related traumatic events in veterans of Operation Desert Storm. Am J Psychiatry
   154(2):173–177, 1997 9016264
Tombaugh TM: The Test of Memory Malingering (TOMM): normative data for cognitively intact and cognitively impaired individuals. Psychol Assess 9:260–268, 1997
   15033228
Vrij A, Mann S: Deceptive responses and detecting deceit, in Malingering and Illness Deception. Edited by Halligan PW, Bass C, Oakley DA. Oxford, UK, Oxford University Press, 2003, pp 348–362

CHAPTER 11

ICD-10, ICD-11, and DSM-5

NEW DEVELOPMENTS AND
THE CROSSWALKS

Andreas Maercker, M.D., Ph.D.
Axel Perkonigg, Ph.D.

THE SEARCH for diagnostic and therapeutic advancements is an international endeavor of relevant professional and interested stakeholders. The *International Statistical Classification of Diseases and Related Health Problems*—currently in its tenth revision (ICD-10; World Health Organization (1992)), with the upcoming revision (ICD-11) expected for 2017—is a major product of these international efforts of psychiatrists and other clinical and research professionals. The ICD's issuing agency, the World Health Organization (WHO), as the directing and coordinating authority for health within the United Nations system, has responsibility for the development of global health standards and for organizing global agreements regarding the definitions of illnesses and diseases (Reed 2010). The organization's constitution describes the WHO's primary tasks as the definition and the naming of diseases and the standardization of diagnostic applications.

In this chapter, we first present a comprehensive overview of WHO's development of the ICD subchapter on stress and trauma disorders. Second, we describe the relevant diagnostic categories from ICD-10 and the planned ICD-11 in more detail. Third, we provide a crosswalk table to compare ICD-10, DSM-5 (American Psychiatric Association 2013), and the planned ICD-11. Finally, we summarize the evidence base for specific treatments for ICD-10 or ICD-11 stress- and trauma-related disorder categories.

DEVELOPMENT OF RELEVANT ICD CHAPTERS

The ICD has a history of more than 150 years. It was developed from the "International List of Causes of Death," edited by the International Statistical Congress in 1900 (this list was later counted as ICD-1). Beginning with the sixth revision in 1948, called the "International List of Diseases and Causes of Death," the WHO (founded in 1946) took charge of this list. Apart from approving the comprehensive list for both morbidity and mortality, WHO's World Health Assembly recommended the adoption of a comprehensive program of international cooperation in the field of vital and health studies. In the ninth edition in 1975, mental health diagnostic categories were modified to include glossaries instead of simply enumerating labels or names of the categories. This change marked the beginning of a movement toward operationalized diagnostic criteria in psychiatry, which was achieved with the publication of DSM-III in 1980 (American Psychiatric Association 1980) and was followed by ICD-10's operationalized research criteria in 1992.

In ICD-10 the diagnostic grouping of reaction to severe stress and adjustment disorders (F43) consists of acute stress reaction (with three subtypes), posttraumatic stress disorder (PTSD), and adjustment disorders (ADs) (with five specific and two residual subtypes). Another relevant category is enduring personality change after catastrophic experience (F62.0), subsumed under disorders of adult personality and behaviour. Relevant diagnostic categories in childhood and adolescence are reactive attachment disorder of childhood (F94.1) and disinhibited attachment disorder of childhood (F94.2), which are placed in the grouping disorders of social functioning with onset specific to childhood and adolescence.

For ICD-11 a working group on disorders specifically associated with stress was established, consisting of 14 members from a number of different continents. The group included psychiatrists, psychologists, and nonspecialists (e.g., nurses, primary care providers); members from minimally resourced countries; and non-English-speaking representatives. This working group assumed a proposed flat, single-level structure for all diagnostic categories (e.g., PTSD, complex PTSD, prolonged grief disorder, AD rather than subtypes) (Maercker et al. 2014). Recent WHO-led research in eight countries showed that clinicians globally have a preference for relatively flat classification systems (Reed et al. 2013). As a result of an intensive process of reviewing the research literature and collecting clinical or field work expertise from around the world, the working group will propose a new and more extensive grouping of the relevant disorders to the governing body of WHO, the World Health Assembly, in 2015. The new subchapter, to be named "Disorders Specifically Associated With Stress," will consist of posttraumatic stress disorder, complex posttraumatic stress disorder, adjustment disorder, prolonged grief disorder, and the two childhood disorders (reactive attachment disorder of childhood and disinhibited attachment disorder of childhood) but will not include the category of acute stress reaction (Maercker et al. 2013). At present, only narrative definitions of these disorders are elaborated for clinical purposes among all WHO member countries. Operationalized criteria for research are not yet available in the ICD-11 Beta Draft but will be elaborated after ICD-11 has been approved by the member countries.

DIAGNOSTIC CATEGORIES IN ICD-10

In this section, we provide the core definitions of the currently existing stress disorders from ICD-10. The original phrasing from World Health Organization (1992) is set off as block quotes, and omissions are marked.

Acute Stress Reaction, ICD-10

> A transient disorder that develops in an individual without any other apparent mental disorder in response to exceptional physical and mental stress and that usually subsides within hours or days. The stressor may be an overwhelming traumatic experience involving serious threat to the security or physical integrity of the individual or of a loved person(s) (e.g., natural catastrophe, accident, battle, criminal assault, rape), or an unusually sudden and threatening change in the social position and/or network of the individual, such as multiple bereavement or domestic fire. The risk of this condition developing is increased if physical exhaustion or organic factors are also present....
>
> The symptoms show great variation but typically they include an initial state of "daze," with some constriction of the field of consciousness and narrowing of attention, inability to comprehend stimuli, and disorientation. This state may be followed either by further withdrawal from the surrounding situation (to the extent of a dissociative stupor—see F44.2), or by agitation and over-activity (Flight reaction or fugue)....
>
> The diagnosis should not be used to cover sudden exacerbations of symptoms in individuals already showing symptoms that fulfill the criteria of any other psychiatric disorder, except for those in the personality disorders section....
>
> Previous labels include: acute crisis reaction, combat fatigue, crisis state, psychic shock.

Posttraumatic Stress Disorder, ICD-10

> The condition arises as a delayed and/or protracted response to a stressful event or situation (either short- or long-lasting) of an exceptional threatening or catastrophic nature, which is likely to cause pervasive distress in almost anyone. Predisposing factors, such as personality traits (e.g., compulsive, asthenic) or

previous history of neurotic illness, may lower the threshold for the development of the syndrome or aggravate its course, but they are neither necessary nor sufficient to explain its occurrence.

Typical features include episodes of repeated reliving of the trauma in intrusive memories ("flashbacks"), dreams or nightmares, occurring against the persisting background of a sense of "numbness" and emotional blunting, detachment from other people, unresponsiveness to surroundings, anhedonia, and avoidance of activities and situations reminiscent of the trauma....

There is usually a state of autonomic hyperarousal with hypervigilance, an enhanced startle reaction, and insomnia. Anxiety and depression are commonly associated with the above symptoms and signs, and suicidal ideation is not infrequent.... The onset follows the trauma with a latency period that may range from a few weeks to months. The course is fluctuating but recovery can be expected in the majority of cases. In a small proportion of cases the condition may follow a chronic course over many years, with eventual transition to an enduring personality change (see F62.0).

Adjustment Disorders, ICD-10

States of subjective distress and emotional disturbance, usually interfering with social functioning and performance, and arising in the period of adaptation to a significant life change or a stressful life event (including the presence or possibility of serious physical illness). The stressor may have affected the integrity of an individual's social network (through bereavement or separation experiences) or the wider system of social supports and values (migration or refugee status), or represented a major developmental transition or crisis (going to school, becoming a parent, failure to attain a cherished personal goal, retirement). The stressor may involve only the individual or also his or her group or community.

Individual predisposition or vulnerability plays an important role in the risk of occurrence and the shaping of the manifestations of adjustment disorders, but it is nevertheless assumed that the condition would not have arisen without the stressor. The manifestations vary, and include depressed mood, anxiety or worry (or mixture of these), a feeling of inability to cope, plan ahead, or continue in the present situation, as well as some degree of disability in the performance of daily routine. Conduct disorders may be an associated feature, particularly in adolescents. The predominant feature may be a brief or prolonged depressive reaction, or a disturbance of other emotions and conduct.

The onset is usually within 1 month of the occurrence of the stressful event or life change, and the duration of symptoms does not usually exceed 6 months, except in the case of prolonged depressive reaction....

Grief reactions of any duration, considered to be abnormal because of their form or content, should be coded as Adjustment Disorder of one of the following Subtypes: brief depressive reaction (not appropriate for bereavement reaction), prolonged depressive reaction, mixed anxiety and depressive reaction, with predominant disturbance of other emotions, with predominant disturbance of conduct, with mixed disturbance of emotions and conduct, or with other specified predominant symptoms.

Previous labels include: culture shock, grief reaction.

Enduring Personality Change After Catastrophic Experience, ICD-10

Enduring personality change may follow the experience of catastrophic stress. The stress must be so extreme that it is unnecessary to consider personal vulnerability in order to explain its profound effect on the personality. Examples include concentration camp experiences, torture, long-lasting disaster, prolonged exposure to life-threatening circumstances (e.g., hostage situations—prolonged captivity with an imminent possibility of being killed). Post-traumatic stress disorder may precede this type of personality change, which may then be seen as a chronic, irreversible sequel of stress disorder.... However, long-term change in personality following short-term exposure to a life-threatening experience such as a car accident should not be included in this category....

In order to make the diagnosis, it is essential to establish the presence of features not previously seen, such as: (a) a hostile or mistrustful attitude towards the world; (b) social withdrawal; (c) feelings of emptiness or hopelessness; (d) a chronic feeling of being "on edge," as if constantly threatened; (e) estrangement. This personality change must have been present for at least 2 years, and should not be attributable to a pre-existing personality disorder or to a mental disorder other than post-traumatic stress disorder.

PROPOSED DIAGNOSTIC CATEGORIES IN ICD-11

In the upcoming ICD-11, not only have the category names and numbers of disorders changed compared with ICD-10, but the definitions will have marked differences, as indicated in the following paragraphs on the specific ICD-11 disorders and the justification for these changes. Additional culture-related features are also provided.

The following short narrative definitions are drawn from the digital publication ICD-11 Beta Draft at the WHO Web site (http://apps.who.int/classifications/icd11, accessed July 31, 2015) and are subject to potential change or refinement in the coming months (see Reed 2010). The relevant disorders are included in the chapter "Mental and Behavioural Disorders" (these disorders are separate from the chapter "Sleep-Wake Disorders" and 23 other chapters dealing with physical health). The "Mental and Behavioural Disorders" chapter contains 19 subchapters, the sixth of which is "Disorders Specifically Associated With Stress."

Posttraumatic Stress Disorder, ICD-11

Post-traumatic stress disorder (PTSD) is a disorder that may develop following exposure to an extremely threatening or horrific event or series of events characterized by reexperiencing the traumatic event or events in the present in the form of vivid intrusive memories, flashbacks, or nightmares, typically accompanied by strong and overwhelming emotions such as fear or horror, and strong physical sensations, avoidance of thoughts and memories of the event or events, or avoidance of activities, situations, or people reminiscent of the event or events, and persistent perceptions of heightened current threat, for example as indicated by hypervigilance or an enhanced startle reaction to stimuli such as unexpected noises. The symptoms must last for at least several weeks and cause significant impairment in functioning.

Rationale for Change From ICD-10 to ICD-11

The most important innovation in ICD-11 involves specifying *core elements* rather than *typical features* of PTSD. Core elements are based on empirical or theoretical grounds and are specific with respect to PTSD by most clearly distinguishing it from other disorders. In contrast, typical features—such as irritability, lack of concentration, or feelings of detachment or estrangement from others—are commonly present but are likely to represent general distress or dysphoria rather than being specific to PTSD (Brewin et al. 2009).

The definition of PTSD requires functional impairment to differentiate it from normal-range reactions to extreme stressors. Furthermore, the time frame requirement is set as a persistent response lasting at least several weeks to an extremely threatening event or series of events. PTSD symptoms arise within 1–6 months after the event. The course of the disorder is often fluctuating (Bryant et al. 2013). Individuals with long-lasting symptoms may eventually develop complex PTSD (described next).

Culture-Related Features

Culturally shaped expressions of PTSD symptoms can include a spiritual component; for example, the sense of heightened current threat may result in distressing dreams that are interpreted as indicating spiritual insecurity or ongoing supernatural powers threatening the person (Hinton et al. 2013). For example, among Indonesian (Aceh) civil war survivors, U.S. American Indian veterans, and Cambodian refugees, nightmares are thought to be important indicators of the person's own spiritual status.

Several other symptoms seem to be prominent features in PTSD in certain cultural settings, partly because they are codified into cultural syndromes or *idioms of distress* (Hinton and Lewis-Fernández 2010). For example, cultural expressions of distress following exposure to trauma may manifest through somatic symptoms such as *ohkumlang* (tiredness) and bodily pain among tortured Bhutanese refugees or symptoms such as possession states among refugees from Guinea-Bissau, Mozambique, Uganda, and Bhutan. Other cultural idioms of distress include *susto* (fright sickness) among Latino populations and *kit chraen* (thinking too much) and *sramay* (flashbacks of past traumas in the form of dreams and imagery that spill over into waking life) in Cambodia (First et al. 2015). Although not equivalent to PTSD symptoms, these manifestations could indicate the presence of traumatization that needs to be looked for in culture-sensitive assessment.

Complex Posttraumatic Stress Disorder, ICD-11

> Complex post-traumatic stress disorder (Complex PTSD) is a disorder that may develop following exposure to an event or series of events of an extreme and prolonged or repetitive nature that is experienced as extremely threatening or horrific and from which escape is difficult or impossible (e.g., torture, slavery, genocide campaigns, prolonged domestic violence, repeated childhood sexual or physical abuse). The disorder is characterized by the core symptoms of PTSD; that is, all diagnostic requirements for PTSD have been met at some point during the course of the disorder. In addition, complex PTSD is characterized by 1) severe and pervasive problems in affect regulation; 2) persistent beliefs about oneself as diminished, defeated or worthless, accompanied by deep and pervasive feelings of shame, guilt or failure related to the stressor; and 3) persistent difficulties in sustaining relationships and in feeling close to others. The disturbance causes significant impairment in personal, family, social, educational, occupational or other important areas of functioning.

Rationale for Change From ICD-10 to ICD-11

Complex PTSD (CPTSD) replaces the ICD-10 category enduring personality change after catastrophic experience, which has failed to attract scientific interest and was not well suited to characterizing disorders arising from prolonged stress in early childhood.

CPTSD and PTSD have in common that their diagnoses are determined by their corresponding symptom profile. This simplifies the task of diagnosis for the clinician by focusing on the target of treatment, namely, symptoms and problems, rather than on trauma history. The CPTSD definition proposes the association of the diagnosis with multiple stressors as a risk factor for the disorder rather than a requirement of it. Thus, CPTSD is determined by the symptom complex rather than by the duration, severity, or number of stressors. However, high probabilities of associations between exposure to sustained traumatic stressors and disturbances in affect, self-concept, and relational difficulties have been supported in the literature (Briere and Rickards 2007).

In addition to the three core features of PTSD (reexperiencing, avoidance, hyperarousal), three additional features apply to CPTSD. These are 1) problems in affect regulation, 2) negative self-concept, and 3) disturbances in relational functioning. These reflect the presence of stressor-induced disturbances that are enduring, persistent, or pervasive in nature and that are not necessarily bound to trauma-related stimuli for their expression.

Problems in affect regulation concern a range of symptoms resulting from difficulties in emotion regulation and can be manifested by heightened emotional reactivity or in the lack of emotions and lapses into dissociative states. Associated behavioral disturbances can include violent outbursts and reckless or self-destructive behavior. Problems with self-concept refer to persistent negative beliefs about oneself as diminished, defeated, or worthless. These beliefs may be accompanied by deep and pervasive feelings of shame, guilt, or failure related to, for example, not having overcome adverse circumstances or not having been able to prevent the suffering of others. Disturbances in relational functioning are exemplified primarily by difficulties in feeling close to others. The person may consistently avoid, deride, or have little interest in relationships and social engagement more generally. Alternatively, there are also persistent difficulties in sustaining relationships.

With respect to other diagnoses, CPTSD can be distinguished from borderline personality disorder (BPD) by the nature of the constellation of symptoms, by differences in the risk for self-harm (Courtois and Ford 2009; Cloitre et al. 2013), and by the type of treatment required for a good outcome. Diagnosis of BPD does not require the presence of a stressor event or the core symptoms of PTSD (Courtois and Ford 2009). BPD is strongly characterized by fear of abandonment, shifting identity, and frequent suicidal behaviors. In CPTSD, the fear of abandonment is not a requirement of the disorder, and self-identity is consistently negative rather than shifting (Cloitre et al. 2011a, 2013). Although suicidal behaviors may be reported, they occur much less frequently in patients with CPTSD than in patients with BPD.

Culture-Related Features

In adults with CPTSD, somatic complaints are frequently present but vary by culture (de Jong et al. 2005). These complaints may partially be associated with previous physical adversities typically co-occurring with prolonged trauma (e.g., inadequate food, clothing, or shelter; experiences of physical punishment, torture, excessive labors, or sexual or other forms of physical exploitation). There are variations in the presentation of the six core domains of CPTSD symptoms by culture (i.e., interpretations and potential spiritual meaning of symptoms) (Hinton et al. 2013). Finally, reporting or assessing CPTSD symptoms can be restricted in trauma survivors because of cultural constraints, particularly among those individuals who have experienced sexual violence. In these cases victims could be extremely reluctant to recount details because their families and society may penalize them if their experiences become known.

Adjustment Disorder, ICD-11

Adjustment disorder is a maladaptive reaction to identifiable psychosocial stressor(s) or life change(s) characterized by preoccupation with the stressor and failure to adapt. The failure to adapt may be manifested by a range of symptoms that interfere with everyday functioning, such as difficulties concentrating or sleep disturbance. Symptoms of anxiety, depression, and impulse control or conduct problems are commonly present and may be the presenting feature. The symptoms emerge within a month of the onset of the stressor(s) and tend to resolve in 6 months unless the stressor persists for a longer duration. In order to be diagnosed, Adjustment disorder must be associated with significant distress and significant impairment in personal, family, social, educational, occupational or other important areas of functioning.

Rationale for Change From ICD-10 to ICD-11

Central to the symptom pattern in AD are preoccupations with the stressor or its consequences, such as excessive worry, recurrent and distressing thoughts about the stressor, or constant rumination about its implications. Symptoms of failure to adapt to the stressor involve those that interfere with everyday functioning, such as difficulties concentrating or sleep disturbance resulting in performance problems at work or school. The symptoms also can be associated with avoidance of stimuli, thoughts, feelings, or discussions associated with the stressor(s) to prevent preoccupation or suffering.

Several studies using the previous ICD-10 AD definition had shown that there is no evidence for the clinical utility of AD subtypes because the characteristic feature is often the mixture of emotional and behavioral symptoms (Strain et al. 1998; Zimmerman et al. 2013). Although internalizing or externalizing symptoms may predominate, in the presenting clinical picture they often coexist. Subtypes are also not helpful in terms of treatment and are not associated with a specific prognosis (Horowitz 2011).

Culture-Related Features

Culture will influence the meaning assigned to the stressor(s), and the meaning in turn will subsequently influence the avoidance (if the meaning is shameful, taboo, etc.) or the sharing of the distress or its hidden quality. For example, imprisonment of a parent in North America is most often a shameful stressor for children and adolescents; however, despite still being a stressor, it can be a source of pride for adolescents whose parents have been imprisoned for political reasons. As another example, the concept of "burnout" could be considered a specific cultural expression of AD related to the workplace. The expression of AD can adopt multiple cultural idioms of distress, which also overlap with those of anxiety disorders (e.g., *ataque de nervios* in Latin America, *latah* in Malaysia). AD has been shown to be a useful concept in different cultural settings (Dobricki et al. 2010).

The stressor may involve only the individual or also his or her group or community. In the latter case, it may affect the integrity of an individual's familial or social network (through bereavement or separation experiences) or the wider system of social supports and values (migration or refugee status).

Prolonged Grief Disorder, ICD-11

Prolonged grief disorder is a disturbance in which, following the death of a partner, parent, child, or other person close to the bereaved, there is persistent and pervasive grief response characterized by longing for the deceased or persistent preoccupation with the deceased accompanied by intense emotional pain (e.g., sadness, guilt, anger, denial, blame, difficulty accepting the death, feeling one has lost a part of one's self, an inability to experience positive mood, emotional numbness, difficulty in engaging with social or other activities). The grief response has persisted for an atypically long period of time following the loss (more than 6 months at a minimum) and clearly exceeds expected social, cultural or religious norms for the individual's culture and context. Grief reactions that have persisted for longer periods that are within a normative period of grieving given the person's cultural and religious context are viewed as normal bereavement responses and are not assigned a diagnosis. The disturbance causes significant impairment in personal, family, social, educational, occupational or other important areas of functioning.

Rationale for Change From ICD-10 to ICD-11

The introduction of prolonged grief disorder (PGD) as a new diagnosis for ICD-11 can be viewed as a response to increasing evidence of a distinct and debilitating condition that is not adequately described by previous ICD diagnoses. Although most people at least partially recover from the acute pain of grief several months following a bereavement, those who continue experiencing severe grief reactions beyond this time frame are likely to have a significant impairment in their general functioning (Shear et al. 2011).

The symptom profile is defined as a severe and persisting (at least over several months) pattern of yearning or longing symptoms for the deceased or a persistent preoccupation with the circumstances of the death. This response may be associated with difficulties accepting the death, feelings of loss of a part of oneself, anger about the loss, guilt or blame regarding the death, or difficulties in engaging with new social or other activities because of the loss. PGD can be diagnosed only if symptoms are still apparent around 6 months after the death and if they markedly interfere with one's capacity to function. In some cultural contexts in which prolonged grieving is normative, it may be more appropriate to assign this diagnosis only after symptoms have persisted for a longer period (e.g., 1 year or even longer).

Culture-Related Features

Mourning shows substantial cultural and developmental variation. A diagnosis of PGD needs to take into account culturally appropriate norms of grieving, and interpretation of prolonged abnormal responses should be made only if the response is aberrant from the cultural norm. For example, Buddhist Cambodians report the need for "merit making" in which the bereaved will continue to focus on the deceased with rituals to facilitate their progress to the next life; it is important not to confuse this practice with excessive preoccupation. In other cultures (e.g., the North American Cree), people will avoid speaking of the deceased for a year after the person's death. Characteristically, there are culture-specific rituals to deal with death and grief or for ceremonies after the death and at anniversaries. The inability or failure to perform these rituals or ceremonies can lead to prolongation of the grief, complications, and guilt. Prolonged grief can also result from the absence of a person's remains so that last rites cannot be performed or a lack of closure due to uncertainty about death, such as a person's disappearance.

A previous proposal for PGD (Prigerson et al. 2009) has been validated across a wide range of cultures, including non-Western settings in China, Iran, Japan, Pakistan, and Rwanda, and has been found to be acceptable cross-culturally (e.g., Lichtenthal et al. 2004; Shear et al. 2011).

Child Stress and Trauma Disorders

The following two diagnostic categories are presented only briefly because these are less relevant to the current book, which relates to adults.

Reactive Attachment Disorder, ICD-11

Reactive attachment disorder is characterized by grossly abnormal attachment behaviours in early childhood, occurring in the context of a history of grossly inadequate child care (e.g., severe neglect, maltreatment, institutional deprivation). Even when an adequate primary caregiver is newly available, the child does not turn to the primary caregiver for comfort, support and nurture, rarely displays security-seeking behaviours towards any adult, and does not respond when comfort is offered. Reactive attachment disorder can only be diagnosed in children, and features of the disorder develop within the first 5 years of life. However, the disorder cannot be diagnosed before the age of 1 year (or a mental age of less than 9 months), when the capacity for selective attachments may not be fully developed, or in the context of Autism spectrum disorder.

Disinhibited Social Engagement Disorder, ICD-11

Disinhibited social engagement disorder is characterized by grossly abnormal social behaviour, occurring in the context of a history of grossly inadequate child care (e.g., severe neglect, institutional deprivation). The child approaches adults indiscriminately, lacks reticence to approach, will go away with unfamiliar adults, and exhibits overly familiar behaviour towards strangers. Disinhibited social engagement disorder can only be diagnosed in children, and features of the disorder develop within the first 5 years of life. However, the disorder cannot be diagnosed before the age of 1 year (or a mental age of less than 9 months), when the capacity for selective attachments may not be fully developed, or in the context of Autism spectrum disorder.

Other Stress and Trauma Disorders

Other Disorders Specifically Associated With Stress, ICD-11

A diagnosis of Other Disorder Specifically Associated With Stress should be used only in cases in which: (a) the clinical presentation does not satisfy the definitional requirements of any of the other disorders in this section or of Acute Stress Reaction; (b) the symptoms are not better explained by another Mental or Behavioral Disorder specified elsewhere in ICD (e.g., a Depressive Disorder or an Anxiety Disorder); (c) the clinical presentation is judged to be a Mental or Behavioral Disorder occurring in specific association with an identifiable stressor. The symptoms cause distress or functional impairment in personal, family, social, educational, occupational or other important areas of functioning.

Disorders Specifically Associated With Stress, Unspecified, ICD-11

This unspecified category is for use when the information in the medical record is insufficient to assign a more specific code and the documentation does not provide additional information to assign a more specific code.

Change Regarding Acute Stress Reaction

The ICD-10 acute stress reaction will no longer be a diagnostic category in ICD-11. In ICD-11, acute stress reaction is being moved to the chapter "Conditions Associated With Psychosocial Circumstances," and the definition from ICD-10 will be unchanged (see "Acute Stress Reaction, ICD-10" above). One major reason for this change is the ambiguity of the definition and diagnostic description as a transient reaction, although the positioning in the ICD-10 chapter on mental and behavioral disorders labeled it as pathology. Although acute stress reaction is similar to PTSD in many respects, and sometimes has been considered as a precursor to PTSD, it differs from PTSD in that greater emphasis is placed on transient dissociative symptoms in acute stress reaction. A review of the available literature on acute stress reaction has cast doubt on the notion that it is a good predictor of later PTSD (Maercker et al. 2013). Another reason for its new position among the conditions associated with psychosocial circumstances is that in some national insurance systems (but not in the United States) acute stress reaction is not recognized as a diagnosis that is covered by health insurance, as it is in many other countries of the world.

CROSSWALK TABLE AND MAIN DIFFERENCES: ICD-10, DSM-5, AND PLANNED ICD-11

Table 11–1 provides a comparison of the ICD-10, DSM-5, and ICD-11 stress and trauma disorders. The main differences or commonalities are recapitulated below.

Acute Stress Disorder/Acute Stress Reaction

What ICD-10 refers to as *acute stress reaction*, DSM-5 lists as *acute stress disorder*. DSM-5 provides an exact time limit of 3 days to 1 month, whereas ICD-10 and ICD-11 refer to a much shorter time: "the symptoms usually begin to diminish after 24–48 hours and are usually minimal after about 3 days." The time required before PTSD is diagnosed has yet to be decided. The symptom descriptions are very similar in all systems. ICD-11 will move this category to the nondisorder chapter "Conditions Associated With Psychosocial Circumstances."

Posttraumatic Stress Disorder

In its criteria for PTSD, DSM-5 explicitly defines potential traumatic events (Criterion A) as actual or threatened death, serious injury, or sexual violence, whereas ICD-10 and ICD-11 present a short (implicit) definition of what constitutes a potential traumatic event. DSM-5 defines four symptom groups (intrusions, avoidance, negative alterations in cognitions and mood, and alterations in arousal and reactivity), whereas the narrative ICD-10 definition includes three (intrusions, avoidance/numbing, hyperarousal). DSM-5 separately defines PTSD for children 6 years and younger, whereas ICD-10 and ICD-11 include paragraphs on childhood symptom presentation but no separate specifier. No specifier "with dissociative symptoms," as used in DSM-5, exists in ICD-10 and ICD-11. The time limits in both diagnostic systems are nearly identical but are less prescriptive in ICD-10 and ICD-11 ("from a few weeks to months…[or] a chronic course over many years").

Enduring Personality Change After Catastrophic Experience/Complex Posttraumatic Stress Disorder

The ICD-10 diagnosis enduring personality change after catastrophic experience and the ICD-11 diagnosis complex posttraumatic stress disorder have no corresponding diagnoses in DSM-5.

TABLE 11–1. ICD-10, DSM-5, and ICD-11 crosswalk

ICD-10		DSM-5		Planned ICD-11
F43.0	Acute stress reaction	308.3	Acute stress disorder	PA32.2[a]	"Acute stress reaction"[b]
			No corresponding diagnosis		
F43.1	Posttraumatic stress disorder	309.81	Posttraumatic stress disorder	6B20	Posttraumatic stress disorder
	No corresponding childhood diagnosis		Posttraumatic stress disorder for children 6 years and younger		*No corresponding childhood diagnosis*
	No additional differentiation		With dissociative symptoms		*No additional differentiation*
			With delayed expression		
F43.2	Adjustment disorders	309.0–4, 9	Adjustment disorders	6B23	Adjustment disorder
	Brief depressive reaction (<1 month)		With depressed mood		*No additional differentiation*
	Prolonged depressive reaction (<2 years)		With anxiety		
	Mixed anxiety and depressive reaction		With mixed anxiety and depression		
	With disturbance of conduct		With disturbance of conduct		
	With mixed disturbance of emotions and conduct		With mixed disturbance of emotions and conduct		
	No corresponding subtype "with anxiety"		*No corresponding depressive subtype differentiation*		

TABLE 11–1.   **ICD-10, DSM-5, and ICD-11 crosswalk *(continued)***

ICD-10		DSM-5	Planned ICD-11	
	309.89	Other specified trauma- and stressor-related disorder Specific reason: Persistent complex bereavement disorder *Also corresponds to persistent complex bereavement disorder in "Conditions for further study"*	6B22	Prolonged grief disorder *Also corresponds to persistent complex bereavement disorder in "Conditions for further study"*
F43.8	Other reactions to severe stress	309.89	Other specified trauma- and stressor-related disorder	6B2Y	Other disorders specifically associated with stress
F62.0	Enduring personality change after catastrophic experience		*No corresponding diagnosis in DSM to either ICD-10 or ICD-11*	6B21	Complex posttraumatic stress disorder
F94.1	Reactive attachment disorder of childhood	313.89	Reactive attachment disorder	6B24	Reactive attachment disorder
F94.2	Disinhibited attachment disorder of childhood	313.89	Disinhibited social engagement disorder	6B25	Disinhibited social engagement disorder

[a]In chapter "Conditions associated with psychosocial circumstances."
[b]Nondisorder phenomenon.

Adjustment Disorder

The descriptions of adjustment disorder are largely analogous in DSM-5 and ICD-10. For ICD-11, major revisions, with positive symptoms (preoccupations, failure to adapt) and an abandonment of subtypes, are suggested.

Prolonged Grief Disorder

For ICD-11, prolonged grief disorder, previously considered an adjustment disorder, is being considered as a new diagnosis in its own right. In DSM-5 it is as before classified as an adjustment disorder when grief reactions exceed what normally might be expected, taking into account cultural, religious, or age-appropriate norms. Furthermore, a patient's disorder is given a code as "other specified trauma- and stressor-related disorder" if symptom characteristics of an adjustment disorder or other trauma- and stressor-related disorder predominate and cause clinically significant distress or impairment but their presentation does not fully meet the criteria for an adjustment or other stressor-related disorder. In this case, the specific reason ("persistent complex bereavement disorder") can be recorded. Additionally, persistent complex bereavement disorder is included, for research purposes, in the DSM-5 chapter "Conditions for Further Study."

Reactive Attachment Disorder, Disinhibited Attachment/Social Engagement Disorder

DSM-5, ICD-10, and ICD-11 do not vary much in their descriptions of reactive attachment disorder and disinhibited attachment (or social engagement) disorder, the two childhood trauma- and stressor-related disorders.

EVIDENCE BASE FOR SPECIFIC TREATMENTS FOR ICD-10 OR ICD-11 DIAGNOSTIC CATEGORIES

One of the reasons for classifying disorders is to facilitate the assignment of appropriate treatments. Therefore, all diagnostic categories in the area of trauma- and stressor-related disorders should help to improve the delivery of specific treatments. WHO referred to available evidence-based treatments when it established new diagnostic categories.

Facilitating treatment includes simplified treatment schemas for conditions of low- and middle-income countries or regions under conflict in the world (Tol et al. 2013). WHO released its Mental Health Gap Action Programme (mh-GAP; World Health Organization 2008) Intervention Guide, which targets acute stress, PTSD, and grief/bereavement and should be easily applicable to the revised diagnoses.

Treatments for PTSD and adjustment disorders are outlined in other chapters of this volume (Chapters 4 and 6, respectively).

For treating PGD, a psychological therapy that strategically targets its symptoms has been shown to alleviate the condition more effectively than unspecific treatments (or those that target adjustment disorder or depression) (Mancini et al. 2012). Several PGD-specific psychotherapies have been developed, including complicated grief treatment, PGD-adapted cognitive-behavioral treatment, structured Internet-based PGD therapy, and self-narrative therapy. Pharmacological approaches are in the process of being researched (Bui et al. 2012).

With regard to CPTSD, it is important to bear in mind that the ICD-11 definition is much narrower than the previous clinical descriptions of "complex trauma" or "complex PTSD" in the literature. Some of the earlier treatment approaches referred to the broader-ranging disorder concepts, but the applicability of these treatments for the new concept has yet to be demonstrated. However, treatments developed for PTSD related to childhood abuse largely apply to the new ICD-11 definition of CPTSD. An expert clinician survey on best practices agreed on several aspects of treatment, including a phase-based therapy and interventions matched to specific symptoms (e.g., emotion regulation strategies, anxiety and stress management, and interpersonal skills) (Cloitre et al. 2011b). The specifically developed treatment model Skills Training in Affective and Interpersonal Regulation (STAIR) proved effective in several clinical trials; it has been refined to STAIR Narrative Story Telling by a second model that focuses on the review and reappraisal of trauma memories (Cloitre et al. 2011a, 2013).

THE FUTURE

DSM-5 and ICD-10 and the upcoming ICD-11 have many features in common but also differ in others. This is true not only for trauma- and stressor-related disorders but for other disorder areas as well. In the United States, as in many other countries, DSM has dominated and still dominates the classification of mental disorders. Clinicians in many other countries have preferred and continue to prefer the ICD. Even in the United States, as a result of a decision by the Centers for Disease Control and Prevention in 2014, use of the ICD classification is on the rise. The information provided about both systems will help all stakeholders and will refine the disciplines involved.

Key Points

- The International Classification of Diseases (ICD) has a history of more than 150 years. It was developed from the 1900 "International List of Causes of Death." Beginning in 1948, the World Health Organization took charge of this classification.

- A new chapter in ICD-11 will be named "Disorders Specifically Associated with Stress."

- The new ICD-11 group will consist of posttraumatic stress disorder, complex posttraumatic stress disorder, adjustment disorder, prolonged grief disorder, and the two childhood disorders reactive attachment disorder and disinhibited attachment disorder.

- The ICD-10 acute stress reaction will no longer be a diagnostic category in ICD-11 and will be moved to the chapter "Conditions Associated With Psychosocial Circumstances" because of the ambiguity of its definition and its transient time course.

- The most important innovation in ICD-11 involves specifying core elements (reexperiencing in the present, avoidance of thoughts and feelings, current sense of threat) rather than typical features of posttraumatic stress disorder.

- The new complex posttraumatic stress disorder replaces the ICD-10 category enduring personality change after catastrophic experience.

- Prolonged grief disorder, previously considered an adjustment disorder, is considered a new diagnosis in its own right in ICD-11.

- A major revision of adjustment disorder in ICD-11 involves increased specification of symptoms and an abandonment of subtypes.

SUGGESTED READINGS

Horowitz MJ: Stress Response Syndromes: PTSD, Grief, Adjustment, and Dissociative Disorders, 5th Edition. Lanham, MD, Jason Aronson, 2011

Maercker A, Znoj H: The younger sibling of PTSD: similarities and differences between complicated grief and posttraumatic stress disorder. Eur J Psychotraumatol 1, 2010

Schulte-Markwort M, Marutt K, Riedesser P: Cross-Walks: ICD-10–DSM IV-TR: A Synopsis of Classifications of Mental Disorders. Cambridge, MA, Hogrefe & Huber, 2003

REFERENCES

American Psychiatric Association: Diagnostic and Statistical Manual of Mental Disorders, 3rd Edition. Washington, DC, American Psychiatric Association, 1980

American Psychiatric Association: Diagnostic and Statistical Manual of Mental Disorders, 5th Edition. Arlington, VA, American Psychiatric Association, 2013

Brewin CR, Lanius RA, Novac A, et al: Reformulating PTSD for DSM-V: life after Criterion A. J Trauma Stress 22(5):366–373, 2009 19743480

Briere J, Rickards S: Self-awareness, affect regulation, and relatedness: differential sequels of childhood versus adult victimization experiences. J Nerv Ment Dis 195(6):497–503, 2007 17568298

Bryant RA, O'Donnell ML, Creamer M, et al: A multisite analysis of the fluctuating course of posttraumatic stress disorder. JAMA Psychiatry 70(8):839–846, 2013 23784521

Bui E, Nadal-Vicens M, Simon NM: Pharmacological approaches to the treatment of complicated grief: rationale and a brief review of the literature. Dialogues Clin Neurosci 14(2):149–157, 2012 22754287

Cloitre M, Cohen LR, Koenen KC: Treating Survivors of Childhood Abuse: Psychotherapy for the Interrupted Life. New York, Guilford, 2011a, 2013

Cloitre M, Courtois CA, Charuvastra A, et al: Treatment of complex PTSD: results of the ISTSS expert clinician survey on best practices. J Trauma Stress 24(6):615–627, 2011b 22147449

Cloitre M, Garvert DW, Brewin CR, et al: Evidence for proposed ICD-11 PTSD and complex PTSD: a latent profile analysis. Eur J Psychotraumatol 4, 2013 23687563

Courtois CA, Ford JD: Treating Complex Traumatic Stress Disorders: An Evidence-Based Guide. New York, Guilford, 2009

de Jong JT, Komproe IH, Spinazzola J, et al: DESNOS in three postconflict settings: assessing cross-cultural construct equivalence. J Trauma Stress 18(1):13–21, 2005 DOI: 10.1002/jts.20005 16281191

Dobricki M, Komproe IH, de Jong JT, et al: Adjustment disorders after severe life-events in four postconflict settings. Soc Psychiatry Psychiatr Epidemiol 45(1):39–46, 2010 DOI: 10.1007/s00127-009-0039-z 19333528

First MB, Reed GM, Hyman SE, et al: The development of the ICD-11 Clinical Descriptions and Diagnostic Guidelines for mental and behavioural disorders. World Psychiatry 14(1):82–90, 2015 25655162

Hinton DE, Lewis-Fernández R: Idioms of distress among trauma survivors: subtypes and clinical utility. Cult Med Psychiatry 34(2):209–218, 2010 20407812

Hinton DE, Field NP, Nickerson A, et al: Dreams of the dead among Cambodian refugees: frequency, phenomenology, and relationship to complicated grief and posttraumatic stress disorder. Death Stud 37(8):750–767, 2013 24521031

Horowitz MJ: Stress Response Syndromes: PTSD, Grief, Adjustment, and Dissociative Disorders, 5th Edition. Lanham, MD, Jason Aronson, 2011

Lichtenthal WG, Cruess DG, Prigerson HG: A case for establishing complicated grief as a distinct mental disorder in DSM-V. Clin Psychol Rev 24(6):637–662, 2004 15385092

Maercker A, Brewin CR, Bryant RA, et al: Diagnosis and classification of disorders specifically associated with stress: proposals for ICD-11. World Psychiatry 12(3):198–206, 2013 24096776

Maercker A, Reed GM, Watts AD, et al: [What do psychologists think about classificatory assessment: WHO-IUPsyS-survey in Germany and Switzerland in preparation for ICD-11]. Psychother Psychosom Med Psychol 64(8):315–321, 2014

Mancini AD, Griffin P, Bonanno GA: Recent trends in the treatment of prolonged grief. Curr Opin Psychiatry 25(1):46–51, 2012 22156937

Prigerson HG, Horowitz MJ, Jacobs SC, et al: Prolonged grief disorder: psychometric validation of criteria proposed for DSM-V and ICD-11. PLoS Med 6(8):e1000121, 2009 19652695

Reed GM: Toward ICD-11: Improving the clinical utility of WHO's International Classification of mental disorders. Prof Psychol Res Pr 41(6):457–464, 2010

Reed GM, Roberts MC, Keeley J, et al: Mental health professionals' natural taxonomies of mental disorders: implications for the clinical utility of the ICD-11 and the DSM-5. J Clin Psychol 69(12):1191–1212, 2013 24122386

Shear MK, Simon N, Wall M, et al: Complicated grief and related bereavement issues for DSM-5. Depress Anxiety 28(2):103–117, 2011 21284063

Strain JJ, Smith GC, Hammer JS, et al: Adjustment disorder: a multisite study of its utilization and interventions in the consultation-liaison psychiatry setting. Gen Hosp Psychiatry 20(3):139–149, 1998 9650031

Tol WA, Barbui C, van Ommeren M: Management of acute stress, PTSD, and bereavement: WHO recommendations. JAMA 310(5):477–478, 2013 23925613

World Health Organization: International Statistical Classification of Diseases and Related Health Problems, 10th Revision. Geneva, World Health Organization, 1992

World Health Organization: mhGAP: Mental Health Gap Action Programme: Scaling Up Care for Mental, Neurological, and Substance Use Disorders. Geneva, Switzerland, World Health Organization, 2008

Zimmerman M, Martinez JH, Dalrymple K, et al: Is the distinction between adjustment disorder with depressed mood and adjustment disorder with mixed anxious and depressed mood valid? Ann Clin Psychiatry 25(4):257–265, 2013 24199215

Epilogue

WITH THE world in considerable chaos and uncertainty, 60 million persons displaced, and war being waged on at least two continents, trauma- and stressor-related disorders abound in these unfortunate communities. Furthermore, the social and cultural stresses of many populations are adding countless concerns and anxieties to millions of persons. Stress is ubiquitous. The question is: when should it be addressed as a disorder? Psychiatry and social science have an important place in attempting to prevent, ameliorate, and manage trauma- and stressor-related disorders. For several generations of DSM taxonomies, some of the trauma- and stressor-related disorders have been poorly served. Despite the fact that the adjustment disorders are the most frequent mental disorder diagnosis in the military and in children, and a common diagnosis in consultation-liaison psychiatry, they have been too frequently regarded as a "wastebasket" diagnosis without sufficient specificity. Some would say they had neither reliability nor validity as a diagnosis. Until DSM-5 placed them in the trauma- and stressor-related category, adjustment disorders were orphaned. It is no exaggeration to point out that all of the disorders now so grouped in the trauma- and stressor-related disorders have been controversial.

It is our hope that with the presentations in this volume, the trauma- and stressor-related disorders will move to a more valid, central focus in psychiatry and in the care of the mentally ill. The American Psychiatric Association, in developing its DSM-5 chapter for these disorders, established a new benchmark for understanding the clinical management of, and the need for additional research on, these entities. Although stress is ubiquitous, it needs to reach a certain level of dysfunction, dysphoria, and interference with the management of life to reach the status of a disorder.

Work will continue to establish the benchmark for the assignment of the designation of disorder for the trauma- and stressor-related genre. Work will also continue to enhance prevention and treatment by focusing on resilience and on the successful management of stress, as well as by developing interventions for acute care and the maintenance of well-being. Furthermore, with advances in technology, our understanding of the biological correlates of stress will be more encompassing, and methods of treatment will be expanded and made more successful in the amelioration of its effects. New targets of treatment will emanate from a greater understanding of the biological basis of stress, as will new methods of prophylaxis from the adversities and comorbidity of stress exposure.

It has been our privilege to present this new and exciting information, and it is our hope that suffering will be lessened and interest in the disorders of stress will be enhanced. Continued research will ultimately lessen the burden imposed by these conditions. We thank our collaborators, whose expertise and devotion to the field have made such salient contributions to our understanding of trauma- and stressor-related disorders. They have pointed us toward enhanced care and needed research and highlighted reasons to be optimistic that we have important tools to help individuals with this group of disorders. Our collaborators working on ICD-11 have also helped to further this goal.

Patricia R. Casey, M.D., F.R.C.Psych.
James J. Strain, M.D.

Index

Page numbers printed in **boldface** *type refer to tables or figures.*